The Biomedical Writer's Handbook

The Biomedical Writer's Handbook

Case-Based Lessons and Applications

Goutham Rao, MD

Jack H. Medalie Professor and Chairman,

Department of Family Medicine and Community Health,

Case Western Reserve University

Editor-in-Chief, Family Practice, Oxford University Press

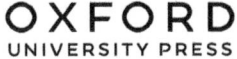

OXFORD
UNIVERSITY PRESS

OXFORD
UNIVERSITY PRESS

Oxford University Press is a department of the University of Oxford.
It furthers the University's objective of excellence in research, scholarship,
and education by publishing worldwide. Oxford is a registered trade mark of
Oxford University Press in the UK and certain other countries.

Published in the United States of America by Oxford University Press
198 Madison Avenue, New York, NY 10016, United States of America.

CIP data is on file at the Library of Congress

This material is not intended to be, and should not be considered, a substitute for medical or other
professional advice. Treatment for the conditions described in this material is highly dependent on
the individual circumstances. And, while this material is designed to offer accurate information with
respect to the subject matter covered and to be current as of the time it was written, research and
knowledge about medical and health issues is constantly evolving and dose schedules for medications
are being revised continually, with new side effects recognized and accounted for regularly. Readers
must therefore always check the product information and clinical procedures with the most up-to-date
published product information and data sheets provided by the manufacturers and the most recent
codes of conduct and safety regulation. The publisher and the authors make no representations or
warranties to readers, express or implied, as to the accuracy or completeness of this material. Without
limiting the foregoing, the publisher and the authors make no representations or warranties as to the
accuracy or efficacy of the drug dosages mentioned in the material. The authors and the publisher do
not accept, and expressly disclaim, any responsibility for any liability, loss or risk that may be claimed or
incurred as a consequence of the use and/ or application of any of the contents of this material.

ISBN 978-0-19-778940-7

DOI: 10.1093/med/9780197789407.001.0001

Printed by Marquis Book Printing, Canada

The manufacturer's authorized representative in the EU for product safety is
Oxford University Press España S.A., Parque Empresarial San Fernando de Henares,
Avenida de Castilla, 2 – 28830 Madrid (www.oup.es/en or product.safety@oup.com).
OUP España S.A. also acts as importer into Spain of products made by the manufacturer.

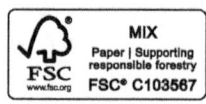

Dedicated to my amazing daughter Lavanya—a future scientist who, at the urging of her dad, is already taking her writing seriously.

Contents

Preface

I completed a fellowship in faculty development in family medicine in Pittsburgh, Pennsylvania, in 1997. In the conference room where fellows met at least once weekly was a whiteboard with a long list of academic projects from current and past fellows that hadn't been completed. These covered a broad range of educational and research topics in family medicine. Included was a proposed new curriculum in alternative and complementary medicine, a number of small projects in sports medicine, and numerous articles of various types. Our beloved fellowship director sometimes pointed to the lengthy list during our weekly meetings to encourage us not to make it longer—in other words, to complete our projects before we graduated. Many prior fellows with incomplete projects would make promises to finish their work at some point, even as they started new jobs in often distant places. Inevitably, their new professional lives would intervene, and they wouldn't revisit the work they had started in Pittsburgh.

What struck me about the whiteboard was that the listed projects were often quite ingenious and that the fellows who started them had already invested a great deal of work. For many research projects, for example, fellows had designed a study protocol, obtained institutional review board approval, implemented study procedures, and even collected data. It was often the last step that was missing—"writing up" the work.

Upon graduation I joined the fellowship program as a faculty member. I taught in a number of different areas. My second book, *Rational Medical Decision Making: A Case-Based Approach*, for example, reflects my strong interest in clinical epidemiology and biostatistics, subjects I taught at the University of Pittsburgh and the University of Chicago for a total of 12 years. The fellows who came after me got a substantial dose of these subjects. Having read a great deal of what they put down on paper, whether it was a case study, the start of an article or abstract, or, in very few cases, a grant application, I worried about the fellows' skills in scientific writing. So, in the year 2000, I added teaching scientific writing to my contributions to the fellowship program.

This book addresses that "last step," expressing important scientific ideas clearly and persuasively. As I discuss in the first chapter, there are few opportunities for biomedical scientists to learn how to write. The book explores the problem and causes of poor scientific writing and introduces readers to a simple paradigm for improving scientific writing. I also cover the most common tasks, such as writing an abstract, that a scientist would need to complete. You'll notice that most of my examples come from the field of primary care research and specifically improving health care delivery for common problems. Being a family physician and a health services researcher in family medicine is part of my core professional identity. You wouldn't want me to include examples from the fields of biochemistry or molecular genetics since they wouldn't be credible. Nevertheless, I believe you can learn something about writing from the examples and exercises in this book, no matter your specific discipline.

I urge you to read the book relatively quickly, perhaps in two or three sittings, and to revisit it often to reenforce the information. You'll also find it helpful to join the Biomedical Writer's Handbook Community online, where you'll find all kinds of helpful information, including opportunities for practice.

I am grateful to the staff at Oxford University Press for allowing me the opportunity to bring my ideas to life, and to all those I've taught over the past 25 years for their insights and suggestions for improvement in my approach. I've learned more from them than they have from me. As you read this book, you may have insights and examples that can also contribute to the field of improving scientific writing. Please share them with our online community.

Goutham Rao, MD
Cleveland, Ohio
February 10, 2025

1

The Challenge of Biomedical Writing

Let's plunge immediately into the problem my book is intended to solve. Start by reading the sentence below:

> Considering that 59% of the control group was correctly predicted, it was concluded that the predictor variables were able to correctly predict membership of the control group, but not able to correctly predict the presently or formerly injured sufferers of trochanteric bursitis.

I plucked the sentence directly from a journal article and changed a few small medical details. You don't benefit from knowing the context in which the sentence appears. One doesn't read isolated sentences from scientific articles. Furthermore, only someone with an interest in trochanteric bursitis would read the paper in which the sentence appears—meaning the sentence might be perfectly understandable under the right circumstances. But is it well-written and does it matter? I argue that it could be better written. I think it's too long and repetitive. Making it shorter, with its point stated more explicitly, would greatly facilitate its clarity. I also believe it matters since the core purpose of written scientific dissemination is to communicate ideas to an audience that is interested in knowing about them. If you can accept this core purpose, the rest of the book should be helpful for you.

Though I'm a medical editor, the sentence above was never officially my duty to fix. But let's consider how that might be done. I mentioned that it is too long. Long sentences can be a strain for readers and the key idea within them can get lost. It's repetitive, with some form of "predict" used four times. What's the basic idea of the sentence? One need not be an expert in trochanteric bursitis nor have access to the entire article to figure out what is being said: The predictor variables are useful in identifying control group members, but not those with trochanteric bursitis. Let's incorporate this basic idea into a new sentence that is shorter and less repetitive: "The predictor variables identified the control group, but not the trochanteric bursitis group accurately."

The revised sentence is just 14 words compared with the original of 42 (three times longer). I am hoping you find it clearer and easier to read overall.

Now imagine that every sentence and passage you read in a journal is written in a way that makes it easy to understand. Wouldn't that be a wonderful thing?

The overall quality of writing in biomedical journals and related publications is indisputably poor, a phenomenon that has been observed for a long time and about which a great deal has been written. In 1911, Andrew MacPhail, editor of the *Canadian Medical Association Journal*, wrote, "There is probably more bad writing in medical journals than in any other kind of periodicals."[1] One hundred and six years later, in the same journal, Roger Collier wrote, "Words matter in science that matters. Far too often, however, the words in medical literature are chosen and arranged without enough care. This leads to confusing, jargon-filled writing that is difficult to read, even for medical researchers."[2] Having taught writing skills to physicians and other biomedical professionals for 25 years and having served as a medical editor of some sort during that time, I have read more than my share of unintelligible scientific prose and don't believe any progress has been made in the quality of writing.

It's not enough, of course, to say that scientific writing is poor; one must identify common problems that can be better defined. In the example above, the original sentence was too long and repetitive, and that made it unclear and hard to understand. Clarity, as we'll discuss, is a significant and widespread problem. Other have observed what's been described as "pompous" or pretentious writing—prose that is unnecessarily complicated, sometimes deliberately so, making it hard to understand. Thorne advised, "Simplicity and clarity are the features of good scientific writing. Clear thought can be expressed clearly, and a man with something of value to say has no need to pad out his account."[3] Many others have called for more clarity and simplicity over the past 100 years.

So why is so much biomedical writing pompous and unclear? There are likely several reasons. First, let's not focus too much on scientists whose first language is not English. An increasing proportion of biomedical literature originates outside of the English-speaking world, and writing clearly in English is not an easy task for many. I have come across many manuscript submissions originating in non-English-speaking countries with excellent ideas expressed in poorly written English. I advise their authors to seek advice from a native English speaker, or else seek the services of a professional English language editor or translator. English remains the paramount

[1] MacPhail A. Style in medical writing. Can Med Assoc J 1911;1:70–73.

[2] Collier R. A call for clarity and quality in medical writing. Can Med Assoc J 2017 Nov 20;189(46):E1407. doi:10.1503/cmaj.171265. PMID: 29158452; PMCID: PMC5698027.

[3] Lock S. *Thorne's better medical writing* (2nd ed.). Pitman Medical Writing, 1977:108–109.

language in scientific literature of all sorts, and I'm deeply sympathetic to those who may speak English very well but struggle with the complexities of our written language.

If we consider only those whose first language is English but who still write poorly in scientific communications, one key reason is that the essential purpose of communicating clearly has been devalued.[4] As a physician-scientist, I know there is enormous pressure to obtain research funding and publish results, especially in high-impact journals. Success has never been defined by how simple or elegant the prose in one's paper is, but whether it has been accepted for publication. Peer reviewers of manuscript submissions focus largely on the quality of the work, including the methods, results, and conclusions, but seldom on the quality of writing, unless it is exceptionally poor, making the entire submission hard to understand. So basically, to many, the quality of writing is an unimportant issue. I think many biomedical writers believe, falsely, that someone—the scientific editor or copyeditor—will sort things out in the end. Given the sheer volume of submissions to any reputable journal and the general hesitancy many editors have to tamper too much with submitted articles, that is an unrealistic expectation.

In addition to devaluing simple, clear writing, some believe that pompous writing persists not because of neglect of the writing process, but because many actually believe it is desirable. The more complicated, pretentious, and lengthy a passage is, often the more sophisticated the author believes it is. So "initiate" appears often in place of "start," and "considerable amounts" appears often in place of "a lot of." The problem persists because junior researchers are encouraged to write pompously by their senior peers, and also to emulate the writing they read in journals.

So a desire to write pompously, perpetuated generation after generation, is a major cause of the problem. But not all biomedical researchers are either prone to or aspire to write pompously. I think there is a much more important cause. I've mentored a large number of practicing physicians and junior researchers for their scholarly projects over the last 25 years. Many started by coming to me with the simple claim, "I've got a great idea for a project that I'd like to tell you about." In many cases the project ideas are genuinely innovative and sound. I next ask for a short, one-page description that includes the rationale for the project and what is to be accomplished, including the outcomes. I usually give such aspiring researchers about a week to send the one-pager to me—but, over the years, only a tiny minority have done so. Why? Is it because they suddenly felt their idea wasn't worthwhile? Did they become

---

[4] Albert T. Why are medical journals so badly written. Med Ed 2004;38:6–8.

so busy that putting together a one-page description wasn't possible? A more detailed example illustrates the core problem. I've changed some of the details to protect my colleague's identity.

About 20 years ago, a close friend and physician colleague of mine (let's call him A.M.) was in the process of completing a graduate degree in public health as a foundation for a career in research. He had been a successful clinician and medical educator for a number of years and excelled in his graduate coursework. The only thing remaining was his thesis paper. The guidelines for the paper were deliberately broad. Students could write about anything related to public health or medicine. Most chose to write a narrative review of timely topics, such as air pollution and its impact on pulmonary disease. No collection of original research data was required. Twenty double-spaced pages was the recommended length.

With 3 months left in his graduate school term, A.M. set out to complete the thesis requirement. Admittedly starting a bit late, he told me he had been distracted by clinical and family responsibilities but had set aside some time each day to do the necessary research and begin writing. I had been teaching writing skills as part of a fellowship program in which he had been enrolled and encouraged him to review some of the materials I had given him a couple of years earlier. Within a week, A.M. had selected a suitable topic: racial and ethnic health disparities in the diagnosis and management of dementia. He began searching for relevant research papers for his narrative review. I checked in with him often, both because I thought I could be helpful in getting him started, and also because he was my friend and I wanted him to succeed. It was very important for him to turn in his paper prior to the end of the term. If he didn't, he would need to enroll in the following fall term just to complete his paper. This would mean paying tuition, which, in the United States, is never a trivial amount.

About a month after starting, A.M. told me he had finalized the list of papers for his review and had begun reading them, making careful notes about key points as he read. He had less than 2 months to go, and I expressed my concern about the limited time remaining. He told me had set aside large "chunks" of time during which he could make a concentrated effort to read and write. This all sounded reasonable to me, but 2 weeks after that, he had made absolutely no progress. He told me he was struggling with an outline for his paper. I sent him a short email describing one broad way to organize it:

1. Discuss the incidence and prevalence of dementia in the United States and worldwide. (500 words)

2. Discuss the benefits of timely diagnosis and potential treatments. (2,500 words)
3. Discuss racial and ethnic disparities in diagnosis and management and the impact upon quality of life of both affected patients and caregivers. (2,500 words)
4. Describe systematic approaches to screening for dementia and tailoring them in a culturally sensitive way for vulnerable groups. (4,500 words)

A.M. thanked me for this basic outline and told me the papers he had retrieved included the necessary information. Time passed quickly, and with a month remaining, he told me he had completed his readings but had made no progress on the paper. A.M. said his clinical practice had gotten busier, his family life had grown more turbulent, and he had lost some precious time due to a nagging back injury. He was nevertheless determined to get the job done but was clearly embarrassed by what he feared I perceived as pure procrastination.

With 1 week remaining prior to the deadline, A.M. came to my office and acknowledged that he hadn't started his paper. He knew that he wasn't going to finish and would need to enroll again in the fall to do so. Thousands of dollars would be wasted.

"I'm quite embarrassed about the whole thing," he told me.

I told him not to be embarrassed but wanted to know what happened. He was bright, hardworking, punctual, and conscientious in so many respects, so his failure to meet a deadline for what I believed was a relatively simple manuscript was perplexing.

"I just don't know how to write," he told me.

And there you have it: a candid confession. He isn't alone. There is little or no training in scientific writing skills in medical school or graduate school curricula. And yet, biomedical researchers are expected to report their ideas and findings clearly and convincingly in manuscripts suitable for publication. I believe scientific writing is a skill to be learned. Neglecting it and still expecting quality written work is like expecting someone to play a musical instrument without any training.

Writing is an important part of training in several non-biomedical professions. Most law school curricula include training in legal writing. Business schools include courses in business writing. So why not scientific writing in medical schools and related institutions? I don't know the answer to that question. I speculate that in medical schools or residency programs, at least, the curricula are deemed already too crowded to add anything more, and writing skills aren't prioritized. Also, designers of medical school curricula can quite accurately claim that the majority of graduates will be practicing clinicians or medical educators who may never engage in endeavors that require scientific writing. In any case, this book is designed to address what I believe is an important need.

I can summarize both the rationale and core principles that underlie *The Biomedical Writer's Handbook* in a few short statements, which should be helpful as you get further into it:

1. Good scientific writing is important to convey important ideas clearly and succinctly.
2. The quality of scientific writing is undermined by a lack of perceived importance, perpetuation of poor writing, and, above all, a lack of training and skills among biomedical researchers.
3. Writing skills are not innate and do not appear spontaneously when needed. Good scientific writing can and needs to be taught.
4. In addition to lots of practice, I believe one can improve writing skills by learning a basic framework and then applying it to important scientific writing tasks.

I've described problems with scientific writing such as a lack of clarity and pompous language. I've also used the term "good scientific writing" several times. But what yardstick should be used to measure good scientific writing? What exactly distinguishes good from poor scientific writing?

For the most part, recommendations for good scientific writing are uniform and include, for example, using simple language. Such recommendations have been made for 100 years or more and are based upon the consensus of journal and book editors and others invested in the quality of writing. They also apply to all fields of writing, from scientific writing to fiction. Recently, there has been an effort to apply science to determine the quality of writing.

Bill Birchard is a journalist and author of the recently published *Writing for Impact: 8 Secrets from Science That Will Fire Up Your Readers' Brains.*[5] Mr. Birchard's recommendations are consistent with others that have been made for generations, such as "Keep it Simple." But he cites evidence for those recommendations based on functional brain imaging studies that show that certain experiences activate certain parts of the brain, including brain centers associated with reward and pleasure. Writing that activates reward centers is assumedly more impactful, more desirable, and of higher quality.

---

[5] Birchard B. *Writing for impact: 8 secrets from science that will fire up your readers' brains.* HarperCollins Leadership, 2023.

Natalie Phillips, a professor of English at Michigan State, used functional magnetic resonance imaging (fMRI) to study the brain's response to reading Jane Austen in two ways: casually and much more closely as one might in preparing for an exam. She found that careful reading of texts activates multiple parts of the brain and reflects coordination of complex cognitive functions, quite distinct from the relatively simple reward-based activation observed during reading for pleasure.[6] While Mr. Birchard's book offers excellent suggestions for writing well (no matter the field), I'm skeptical that good scientific writing can be accurately identified by its impact upon reward centers in fMRI studies. I also don't associate reading scientific prose with reward or pleasure. Yes, like you, I do have a few colleagues who pick up a journal article and read it for the joy of it, but most of us don't. What drives our reading is either curiosity or necessity. Reward, from the standpoint of activation of brain centers, doesn't seem like the right metric for assessing scientific writing.

Furthermore, serious doubts have been raised about the reliability of fMRI studies to assess the impact on the brain of completing specific tasks, including by investigators at Duke who have been leaders in the field for many years.[7]

If the primary aim of scientific communication is for others to understand your work, ease of understanding ought to be the primary measure by which we measure the quality of writing. Don't worry about whether your writing activates reward centers in the brain; worry about whether what you write is easily understood. If you accept this, there are well-established measures of understandability, or readability. The Flesch Reading Ease and the related Flesch–Kinkaid Grade Level tests were developed within the U.S. Navy 50 years ago and have since been applied to all sorts of writing to assess its readability.[8] The score relies on the well-established and intuitively obvious finding that short sentences, fewer words, and simple words are easier to understand than longer, more wordy sentences and more complex words. The Flesch score is a simple calculation based on sentence length/number of words per sentence and the number of syllables per word. While it cannot capture all the nuances that distinguish between easily understood and poorly

[6] This is your brain on Jane Austen, and Stanford researchers are taking notes. https://arts.stanford.edu/this-is-your-brain-on-jane-austen-and-stanford-researchers-are-taking-notes/. Accessed February 5, 2024.

[7] Elliott ML, Knodt AR, Ireland D, et al. What is the test-retest reliability of common task-functional MRI measures? New empirical evidence and a meta-analysis. Psychol Sci 2020 Jul;31(7):792–806. doi:10.1177/0956797620916786. Epub 2020 Jun 3. PMID: 32489141; PMCID: PMC7370246.epu

[8] Kincaid JP, Fishburne RP, Rogers RL, Chissom BS. *Derivation of new readability formulas (automated readability index, fog count, and Flesch reading ease formula) for Navy enlisted personnel.* Research Branch Report 8–75. Chief of Naval Technical Training, Naval Air Station Memphis, 1975.

understood writing, and therefore good and poor writing, it is still a useful rough measure that can be applied to assess and improve your own writing.

Now that we've discussed the principles underlying this book and have at least a good notion of what good scientific writing is, it's time to discuss a relatively simple paradigm that takes advantage of these principles, research findings, and measures of readability that will help you improve your scientific writing.

My own background will be useful to you as you make your way through the book. In addition to being a writing instructor for many years, I'm a proud family physician and established health services researcher. I mostly studied how to improve primary care for common chronic illnesses, especially obesity, diabetes, hypertension, and other cardiovascular risks. You'll find that the majority of examples I use reflect this background. I've stuck with what I know to make my examples as credible as possible. Your background might be quite different from mine. I've tried to keep the examples as simple as possible so that they can be understood by the broad audience for this book. Also, I think that working your way through the examples I provide will help you become a better biomedical writer, no matter your specific field.

2
The 5Cs

If you agree or mostly agree that ease of understanding should be the primary measure by which the quality of scientific writing is judged, we need a way to make scientific writing as easy to read as possible. From the preceding chapter, you've likely already gathered a few common and useful recommendations— avoid jargon; use simple words; avoid redundancy and lengthy sentences. As noted, guidance for what is good scientific writing is largely uniform. A framework to summarize this guidance is useful, not only as you begin to write, but also as you revise what you've written.

Both clinical medicine and research are full of frameworks designed to help us better understand a process, symptom, or disease, or to remind us about what is important. Medical students, for example, are taught to complete a review of systems for pulmonary diseases for a patient presenting with cough or shortness of breath. This includes a set of questions to gather useful information in making a diagnosis and helps them to gather all relevant information systematically. Simultaneously, students learn about underlying causes of common symptoms such as cough. The review of systems helps them link the information they gather to potential underlying causes. Similarly, the health services research world in which I live is full of frameworks for implementing innovations or improvements to care. There are so many such frameworks and they have been used and studied so often that "implementation science" has emerged as a distinct and important discipline. Implementation science frameworks help us incorporate improvements or innovations into patient care in a systematic way and are also used to evaluate progress and success in implementation.

I developed the 5Cs framework more than 20 years ago to emphasize what is important in the quality of scientific writing, to increase self-awareness of one's writing, and as a tool for revising or editing scientific prose. I didn't pull it out of thin air; it's based on the collective wisdom of experts in scientific writing, a survey of common problems and challenges, and a very famous book. Note that there are several paradigms for sound technical or scientific writing, including others titled the "5Cs."[1] Many of these are similar to each

[1] https://www.sparrowconnected.com/blog/5c-of-effective-written-communication-0. Accessed September 5, 2024.

other and to mine, especially one described by Royce Kimmons.[2] While the 5Cs is a common organizational framework for sound scientific writing, the details of the 5Cs and how to implement them are the focus of this book.

I believe all of us who have developed frameworks for writing principles are indebted to Professor William Strunk Jr., whose short book *The Elements of Style* was first published more than 100 years ago to help Cornell University students improve their writing.[3] It has sold more than 10 million copies since, and even as of January 19, 2024, was the sixth best-selling writing skills book on Amazon.com! The book has changed very little over the course of several editions. The *New York Times* has described it as timeless. Its elegant simplicity as a tool to improve writing is unmatched. There are just 11 rules for punctuation and grammar; 11 principles of writing; 11 matters of form; and 21 reminders for better style. I'm a great admirer of the book and have read it many times. The 5Cs framework, though intended for scientific writing, adopts several of Professor Strunk's principles to construct what I hope will be useful for you in both identifying problems in scientific writing and improving it.

The 5Cs are *conciseness, clarity, cogency, commonness,* and *consistency.* I'll explain each of these in detail as well as how to achieve them. They are interrelated and overlapping; conciseness can bring clarity, for example. Learning and applying these five principles separately, however, provides a systematic stepwise approach to improving your writing. It's easier to make a paragraph more concise, then clearer, and then more cogent, for example, than trying to accomplish all these things at once.

Conciseness

The *Oxford Learner's Dictionary* defines conciseness as "the quality of giving only the information that is necessary and important, using few words."[4] You could argue that the word "brevity," which has largely the same meaning, is more concise than conciseness; pity it doesn't begin with the letter "c."

In my many years of reviewing and editing manuscripts and helping others write, this is the principle that biomedical writers are most likely to violate. They simply write too much. Often they don't realize that they have written too much, but sometimes they consciously use too many words, mistakenly

---

[2] https://edtechbooks.org/rapidwriting/5Cs?format=ms_word. Accessed September 5, 2024.
[3] Strunk W Jr., White EB. *The elements of style* (4th ed.). Longman, 2000.
[4] https://www.oxfordlearnersdictionaries.com/us/definition/english/conciseness. Accessed August 3, 2023.

believing this will distinguish their work in some way, perhaps making it seem more sophisticated.

Professor Strunk emphasizes conciseness throughout *The Elements of Style* with the powerful instruction, "Omit needless words!" There are several reasons why conciseness is important:

1. *Space is limited*: Even in the era of open access journals and online publications, most publications have strict page limits. Manuscripts or proposals that exceed these are quickly sent back for revision or are rejected outright (grant submissions, for example). Of course you'd like to include all the information that's important, but you must do so in a way that respects length limitations.

2. *Readers' time is limited*: Less obvious is the fact that readers of biomedical works have limits on how much they are able or willing to read. The average person reads general text at roughly 238 words per minute.[5] The rate for scientific or technical manuscripts, as you can imagine, is far slower: just 75 words a minute.[6] The stuff we write is typically dense with complex information that requires a great deal of thinking as we read. At that rate, the time required to read a manuscript of 3,000 words is 40 minutes; cut it down to 2,000 words and the time is 27 minutes. Thirteen free minutes is enough time to complete clinical documentation for one patient, begin and partly read another manuscript, or enjoy a cup of coffee. Conciseness, therefore, is greatly appreciated by the readers of your work.

3. *Concise writing is quality writing*: Unnecessary words come in many different forms. Imprecise sentences are often lengthy. Flowery language or jargon also makes manuscripts unnecessarily expansive. Omit needless words and you will not only be doing the editors and readers a service but will also improve the quality of your work.

4. *Conciseness is stylish and elegant*: Embrace it. As Hemingway advised us, "Use short sentences."[7] We should all follow his advice no matter what we're writing. Being concise will make your writing less muddy

[5] Brysbaert M. How many words do we read per minute? A review and meta-analysis of reading rate. J Mem Language 2019;109. https://doi.org/10.1016/j.jml.2019.104047

[6] https://wordsrated.com/reading-speed-statistics/#:~:text=Average%20reading%20speed%20by%20p age&text=For%20technical%20material%2C%20the%20average,to%2075%20words%20per%20minute. Accessed August 6, 2023.

[7] Modesitt SC, Havrilesky LJ, Previs RA, et al. Ridiculously good writing: How to write like a pro and publish like a boss. Gynecol Oncol Rep 2022 Jun 10;42:101024. doi:10.1016/j.gore.2022.101024. PMID: 35719321; PMCID: PMC9204657.

and more focused and will make you appear sharp and committed to reaching as many readers with your work as possible.

If I've sold you on the importance of conciseness, let's look at one example. As with all the examples from this book, I've taken it directly from a published paper but have deliberately not included the authors' identity or the citation. Conciseness is the responsibility of both the authors and the editors of a manuscript. Unfortunately, an unnecessarily lengthy passage often slips through the cracks and need not reflect the quality of the journal or its editing process, the caliber of the writer, or, of course, the value of the underlying work.

Read this sentence a couple of times:

Despite the prevalence of these problems of high burnout and low employee engagement and widespread belief that they beget turnover, there remains little published research evidence of a relationship between burnout or engagement and turnover. (36 words)

Did you understand it immediately? I have a role in my hospital titled "chief clinician experience officer" (called "wellness officer" in many institutions) and stay abreast of literature on burnout and engagement among health care professionals, so I had no difficulty understanding the sentence. Nevertheless, I think it's too long, and I think some of you might find yourself reading it twice or at least going back to the first part of the sentence to understand it better. Here is my revised version:

Though turnover is widely believed to result from high burnout and low engagement, little research supports the relationship. (18 words)

The new sentence is half as long. Some of the trimming is easy to accomplish. "The prevalence of these problems of high burnout and low employee engagement" is essentially the same thing as "high burnout and low employee engagement," with "the prevalence of these problems" being unnecessary. "Little published research evidence" is essentially the same thing as "little research." "Turnover" is the focus of the sentence and should be put up front. It's a perfectly good noun that stands on its own, with no need to use "beget" turnover. "Burnout and engagement" are mentioned twice unnecessarily; "supports the relationship" is a more concise way of making the point. You may have come up with other ways of making the sentence more concise while retaining its meaning.

Of course, applying the principle of conciseness takes practice. Experienced writers and editors can draw upon their considerable knowledge of style and usage to trim passages effectively, but how can you make your own writing more concise?

We are all guilty of writing passages that are too long, but because we have written them, we may find them easy to understand and appropriate in length. Trimming one's own writing, therefore, may seem difficult. Furthermore, most biomedical writers, especially those who are less experienced, don't have the knowledge and skills needed to easily rephrase lengthy passages based on their experience reading needless words or phrases. This book is all about using shortcuts to achieving better writing. So here is a four-step process you can follow:

1. Once you've completed a paper, grant, or any other writing related to your profession, read it over carefully and identify passages and paragraphs you believe might be too long. Don't worry about whether they are clear (since wordiness and lack of clarity are often distinct). Just look for parts of your piece you worry might strain the reader because of their length. In a typical page of 500 words, identify a minimum of two passages of this type.
2. Highlight the target passage in Microsoft Word or other word processing program. Microsoft Word will automatically calculate the number of words in the passage. Read the passage a few times. Ask yourself if each word or phrase is necessary to capture the needed meaning.
3. Aim to trim the passage by a third to start. For example, if the target passage is 50 words, try to eliminate 16 or 17 words. Benjamin Dreyer, in his outstanding *Dreyer's English*,[8] identifies a number of useful targets in his chapter entitled "Trimmables." In Table 2.1 I've listed a few that I've seen often in biomedical literature, each followed by the recommended trimmed version.
4. Read the trimmed passage a few times, then read the original passage. Does the revised passage capture the entire intended meaning of the original? If the answer is yes, you can try trimming a few more words or move on. If not, you can either add back parts you believe are important or try trimming the original in other ways.

There is no right or wrong way to go about this process, but I strongly believe everyone ought to do it with all of their writing. The more practice you

---

[8] Dreyer B. *Dreyer's English: An utterly correct guide to clarity and style*. Random House, 2019:242–251.

Table 2.1 Example of Phrases to Shorten

End result → result
Exact same → same
Final outcome → outcome
Merge together → merge
HIV virus → HIV
Join together → join
Daily (or monthly, annually, hourly, etc.) basis → daily
Interdependent upon each other → interdependent
Last of all → last
Mutual cooperation → cooperation
Reason why → reason
Short in length → short
Surrounded on all sides → surrounded
Usual custom → custom

get, the easier it will be become, and your writing will gradually become more concise so that there will be fewer passages to trim.

Let's consider an example. Dr. A has written the following passages as part of a grant application on improving quality of care for diabetes:

> *So, based on the prior work we have completed, as well as the prior study by Benham et al., we believe there is an obvious gap in evidence about the unknown effectiveness of continuous glucose monitors (CGMs). It is unclear if these devices increase self-motivation to improve self-care for diabetes, or if they provide useful data for meaningful adjustments to treatment by physicians and others who provide care for patients with diabetes.* (72 words)

Dr. A is constrained by strict page limits for her grant application. The passage above is part of the background section, and she needs to reserve most of the space for outlining her research plan. She has identified the passage above as prime for trimming. She reads it a few times. Her initial goal is a revised passage of roughly 48 words.

She thinks about each word and phrase carefully and draws the following conclusions:

- Isn't "prior work we have completed" just "our prior work"?
- Is "we believe" necessary? After all, we're the ones submitting the application, so by definition it includes what we believe.

- "Self-motivation" and "self-care" seem redundant, as do "useful" and "meaningful."
- "Who provide care for patients with diabetes" seems completely unnecessary since the grant application is about diabetes.

She ponders these potentially unnecessary phrases for a few moments and then starts her rewrite:

Based on our prior work and that of Benham et al., there is an obvious gap in evidence about the unknown effectiveness of continuous glucose monitors (CGMs). It is unclear if these devices improve self-care or provide data useful for treatment adjustments. (41 words)

Dr. A is quite pleased with her trimming: She has cut down the original passage by well over a third, more than her original goal. She reads the original and revised passages a few times and concludes that the revised passage captures all that she originally intended. But she thinks she may be able to do even better. "There is an obvious gap in evidence about the unknown effectiveness of continuous glucose monitors" seems like a good target for further trimming. "An obvious gap in evidence about the unknown effectiveness" is awkward and lengthy, and "a gap in evidence" refers, by definition, to something unknown.

Dr. A writes:

Based on our prior work and that of Benham et al., the effectiveness of continuous glucose monitors (CGMs) is unknown. It is unclear if these devices improve self-care or provide useful data for treatment adjustments. (35 words)

Dr. A believes she has done well and rereads the revised passage and the original a few times. The phrases "is unknown" and "It is unclear" stand out to her as redundant. She takes an ambitious step, combining the two sentences into one:

Based on our prior work and that of Benham et al., it is unclear if continuous glucose monitors (CGMs) improve self-care or provide useful data for treatment adjustments. (28 words)

Dr. A's final revised passage is just a bit over a third as long as her original—quite a dramatic trimming, resulting in a passage that is not only more concise but also simple and elegant. Being concise requires being very conscious about one's own writing both when writing a piece for the first time and when revising it. As I mentioned, it takes considerable practice.

Clarity

Like conciseness, clarity is an important challenge in scientific writing. Some define clarity simply as the ease with which writing can be understood. Others use the word to encompass many aspects of writing, such as avoiding jargon and being concise. In our everyday lives as readers and writers of scientific prose, clarity or a lack of clarity is often obvious. A passage is unclear if it is poorly written or unclear to an individual due to his or her own personal limitations in understanding it. I offer my own definition below only because it fits nicely in the overall 5Cs paradigm:

> *Scientific writing is clear if the meaning intended by the author matches the understanding of the reader after he or she has read it once. Scientific writing is unclear if the reader doesn't understand the intended meaning after he or she has read it once.*

But what exactly makes writing unclear? Intended meanings can be misunderstood for many reasons, including use of unfamiliar jargon or simple grammatical errors. Those are easily fixable problems. Among Professor Strunk's rules are four I categorize under clarity. We'll get to these as we explore some examples.

Unclear scientific writing isn't hard to find, so I did a little experiment to show just how common it is even in the best journals. Much of my work as a health services researcher deals with obesity and diabetes, so I punched in "diabetes" in the search field in PubMed and filtered results for randomized controlled trials and those available in full-text form free of charge so you can duplicate my search if you wish to. I did this to show you that unclear writing isn't rare, and that I haven't chosen a few passages from obscure journals that I've found by carefully looking over journals over the course of years.

Our first example comes from the first paper retrieved from the list:

> *In the sulfonylurea–insulin group, the significant reduction of 25% in the risk of microvascular disease that was observed during the interventional trial in the intensive-therapy group was sustained throughout the post-trial period, despite the rapid convergence of glycated hemoglobin levels in the two groups*

and a similar use of glucose-lowering therapies, and the reduction in the risk of any diabetes-related end point was also sustained.

Did you understand it after reading it once? You may have, but it should also be obvious that the example is a very long sentence—65 words. There are no clear guidelines for the length of sentences in scientific prose, but 20 words is considered to be a reasonable maximum length for scientific materials intended for the general public.[9] Our first example illustrates one of Professor Strunk's important rules to promote clarity: Avoid overlong sentences. Of course, conciseness is related to overlong sentences, but short sentences don't guarantee conciseness, since you may have too many short sentences. How overlong sentences compromise clarity isn't hard to figure out. By the time you've gotten to the end of a very long sentence, you may have either forgotten or are unable to integrate what was at the beginning. Short sentences are easier to understand.

So, how might we edit the sentence above? Don't worry about conciseness for now (which is also a problem with the sentence). Clarity can be improved quite simply by breaking up the single 65-word sentence into three and reorganizing a bit:

In the sulfonylurea–insulin group, the significant reduction of 25% in the risk of microvascular disease that was observed during the interventional trial in the intensive-therapy group was sustained throughout the post-trial period. The reduction was observed despite the rapid convergence of glycated hemoglobin levels in the two groups and a similar use of glucose-lowering therapies. The reduction in the risk of any diabetes-related end point was also sustained.

I've actually added words to the excerpt. The first sentence is still 33 words long, but there is some medical jargon that is difficult to avoid unless one tries to make the sentence more concise (e.g., taking out "that was observed," which is unnecessary). I hope you find the three shorter sentences easier to understand than the single long one.

Here are some tips to improve clarity by avoiding overlong sentences:

1. Try to limit sentences to roughly 20 words, unless they include longer technical or scientific terms, in which case 30 words is reasonable.

---

[9] Matthews N, Folivi F. Omit needless words: Sentence length perception. PLoS One 2023 Feb 24;18(2):e0282146. doi:10.1371/journal.pone.0282146. PMID: 36827285; PMCID: PMC9955962.

2. Once you've completed a piece, look for overlong sentences. You can easily find their length in Microsoft Word or another program. Break them up into two or three (or even sometimes four) short sentences. You can achieve this by looking for natural breaks in the original sentences. Above, for example, "risk reduction . . . post-trial period" is an important self-contained idea that deserves its own sentence.

3. You may need a couple of additional connecting words as you break up a sentence, just as I have used "The reduction was observed" above.

Now let's turn to another problem that compromises clarity. First, we need to define a broad category of words and phrases known as *modifiers*. A modifier simply enhances the meaning of a sentence. In other words, a sentence may be clear and meaningful without a modifier, but more information is provided when a modifier is included. There are all sorts of modifiers, including clauses with adverbs or adjectives. Consider these examples:

The second assay, which had been carried out in 2022, showed negative results.

In this sentence the clause "which had been carried out in 2022" modifies the "the second assay."

Consider another example:

Because some research subjects arrived too late, their data were not included.

The clause "because some research subjects arrived too late" is known as an adverbial modifying phrase that provides an explanation for why data from some subjects were not included.

Careless use of modifiers creates problems of clarity. The "dangling modifier" is well known in writing circles as a common problem and is the subject of many humorous examples. Here are a few:

After discussing the new software updates, the original equipment stayed in place.

It's easy enough to figure out what is intended, but the problem is that the modifier "After discussing the new software updates" modifies the original equipment, which is not the correct subject: Equipment doesn't usually discuss anything, including software updates. The modifier is said to be *dangling* since the word or phrase it is intended to modify is missing—it's likely the people who discussed the software updates. We can rewrite the sentence as follows:

After we discussed the new software updates, the original equipment stayed in place.

or

After discussing the new software updates, we left the original equipment in place.

Modifiers can also be included but misplaced. Here is an example of a misplaced modifier:

The research team thought about throwing a party for the students while they analyzed data from the previous week.

Doesn't sound like it would be a great time to have a party for the students, does it? Who would want to party while analyzing data? Jokes aside, the intended meaning may be clear, but the sentence is incorrect since the modifier is in the wrong place. Here is a corrected sentence:

While they analyzed data from the previous week, the research team thought about throwing a party for the students.

Finally, let's consider ambiguous modifiers, also known as "squinting" modifiers. Here is an example:

Explaining the consent process clearly makes recruitment success more likely.

The modifier "clearly" is ambiguous because (1) it could modify "explaining the consent process," meaning the consent process is described well or (2) it could modify "makes recruitment success more likely," meaning it is apparent or obvious that recruitment would benefit. Let's say the intent was to modify recruitment success. We could rewrite the sentence as follows:

Explaining the consent process will clearly make recruitment success more likely.

You might wonder at this point if bringing clarity to writing by avoiding problems with modifiers really matters. After all, in the examples above (perhaps with the exception of the last one), the sentences are relatively simple and the intent of the writer is clear. Why dwell on what you might believe is a simple grammatical issue that can be easily corrected by software? Unfortunately, the intent of the writer (such as in the last example) can be unclear to differing degrees depending upon who is reading a passage. Here's a sentence from the same PubMed search I described earlier:

> *After calling for subjects entering the research project, 24 females were randomly (Simple) selected and then randomly divided into two equal groups: control and experimental (N = 12).*

This sentence has a relatively straightforward dangling modifier—it sounds like the "24 females" called for "subjects entering the research project." You are likely familiar with research and the scientific process, so it was probably easy for you to understand the sentence as it was intended. However, that may not be the case for someone with less experience, including those who are just starting to read research papers. A missing modifier can be added:

> *After we called for subjects entering the research project, 24 females were randomly (Simple) selected and then randomly divided into two equal groups: control and experimental (N =12).*

Consider another example:

> *Briefly, patients were randomised 1:1, stratified in blocks by sex, age, known diabetes duration and urinary albumin excretion rate (<100 mg/day vs >100 mg/day) using sealed envelopes, to receive either conventional multifactorial treatment with treatment goals at all times according to existing national guidelines or to receive intensified, multifactorial treatment targeting co-existing risk factors for late diabetic complications.*

This sentence has a relatively straightforward misplaced modifier. Randomization took place using sealed envelopes, but a reader might interpret that "using sealed envelopes" modifies "urinary albumin excretion rate." In other words, somehow urinary albumin excretion with sealed envelopes is a characteristic upon which to base randomization. Such an interpretation is, of course, unlikely, given the overall context and familiarity with research methods that many readers, though not all, might have. Your goal should be to make your writing clear to everyone. A better sentence begins with:

Briefly, using sealed envelopes we randomized patients 1:1 …

Now here's an example that may be more ambiguous even for an experienced reader, especially without lots of context:

Randomization will be stratified by the TCM Skill Training Centre.

Is the TCM Skill Training Centre the entity that will perform the stratified randomization? Or is the TCM Skill Training Centre the unit of randomization? Reading the rest of the methods section of the paper would provide greater context that would make it clear that the former is what is intended. However, especially if you read that sentence quickly, no matter your experience in reading scientific articles, you might think the latter is what was intended. The sentence can be simply rewritten as:

The TCM Skill Training Centre will complete stratified randomization (of patients).

Avoiding dangling, misplaced, or squinting modifiers is included in Professor Strunk's advice to keep related words together, whether it be to avoid misplaced modifiers or not. He offers the following examples:

This is a portrait of Benjamin Harrison, grandson of William Henry Harrison, who became President in 1889.

So who became President in 1889: William Henry Harrison or Benjamin Harrison? Clarity can be achieved with two sentences:

This is a portrait of Benjamin Harrison, who became President in 1889. He was the grandson of William Henry Harrison.

Or, as suggested by Professor Strunk:

This is a portrait of Benjamin Harrison, grandson of William Henry Harrison. He became President in 1889.

Essentially, the sound advice to keep related words together and to be conscious of dangling, misplaced, and squinting modifiers will help improve the clarity of your writing. I can't suggest any trick or algorithm to identify clarity problems related to the order or "missingness" of words such as in the examples above. A good general approach would be to read each paragraph you've written and to underline any sentences you believe could be interpreted in another way, especially with clauses intended to modify or add detail to a description. Then go back and add subjects, phrases, or split sentences to clear things up.

A final suggestion to enhance clarity is Professor Strunk's advice to "express co-ordinate ideas in similar form," which is known as the principle of parallel construction. According to Strunk, "the likeness of form enables the reader to more readily recognize the likeness of content and function" and therefore enhances clarity. He goes on to insist that unskilled writers believe that constantly varying the form of expression is necessary. The classic example he provides is:

> *Formerly science was taught by the textbook method, while now the laboratory method is employed.*

A consistent form of expression makes the writer seem more committed to one form of expression and also makes the sentence clearer:

> *Formerly science was taught by the textbook method; now it is taught by the laboratory method.*

This basic writing principle is violated often in biomedical literature, including in the search for diabetes articles I carried out:

> *Energy metabolism objectives assessed the effects of tirzepatide versus placebo and semaglutide on body weight, body composition, fasting appetite, and energy intake during ad libitum lunch.*

The outcomes of tirzepatide, placebo, and semaglutide are body weight, body composition, fasting appetite, and the last, which is expressed in a different form than the first three. While the sentence may be comprehensible, it would be clearer and easier to read as follows:

> *Energy metabolism objectives assessed the effects of tirzepatide versus placebo and semaglutide on body weight, body composition, fasting appetite, and ad libitum lunch energy intake.*

"Ad libitum lunch energy intake" is more similar in form to the other three outcomes than "energy intake during ad libitum lunch," which seems like a much more complex term or outcome that may cause the reader to revisit the sentence, a sign of a lack of clarity.

My best advice is for you is to keep the principle of expressing co-ordinate ideas in similar form in mind as you write, and immediately abandon the belief that varying forms is necessary or makes your writing more sophisticated.

Cogency

In my view, while all 5Cs are interrelated, conciseness and clarity are paramount. Cogency is also important and can be defined as referring to something that is expressed clearly and persuasively—in other words, convincingly. I chose "cogency" instead of "convincing" since the other four Cs are nouns and convincing is an adjective. The noun form of convincing, convincingness, is very uncommonly used and sounds neither concise, clear, nor cogent itself.

One of Professor Strunk's rules is to use definite, concrete language. One form of violation of this rule is very common in the biomedical literature. Consider this especially glaring example:

> *Alternatively, and in our view, far more likely, it is possible that if edema forms during the obstruction, it may be roentgenologically masked, perhaps by increases in lung volume.*

Given the full context in which the sentence appears, the sentence may be reasonably well understood. However, the author includes so many expressions of doubt or uncertainty that it's unclear what he or she actually believes. This is known as "hedging," and when it's excessive, it zaps all the power out of a sentence or passage and makes it less cogent. Hedges in the sentence above include "in our view," "far mor likely," "it is possible," "if edema forms," "it may be," and "perhaps." Six hedges in one sentence! Including far fewer hedges makes the sentence more persuasive. There is nothing wrong with expressing uncertainty, especially in scientific literature, but sometimes hedging becomes a tool to cover all bases or remain noncommittal to such an extent that the sentence has no meaning.

Here's another example:

> *It is possible that some infections may take place among some patients in particular circumstances spontaneously.*

Four hedges here: "It is possible," "may take place," "some patients," and "in particular circumstances."

Imagine that you show up at an airport and ask the counter attendant if your flight is late and he responds, "It's possible in some circumstances that your flight may be late." Surely you wouldn't be pleased with such a response! As readers, we are naturally averse to hedging because all the doubt makes us unsure about what we are supposed to take away from a sentence or passage.

Here's an example from the diabetes search:

Our study suggests that the beneficial effects of FMT may not be mediated solely through improvements in glycemic response.

Even though there are only two hedges in this sentence—"Our study suggests" and "may not be mediated"—some of the sentence's cogency is lost. "Our study suggests" is an unnecessary hedge that makes the study findings less certain. As a rule, I advise you to include no more than one hedge in a sentence, two if you must.

Fixing hedging is relatively straightforward. In addition to being aware of it as you write, go back through your writing and look for hedges that are common in the biomedical literature, such as "may," "it is possible," "might," "suggests," "implies," "under some circumstances," and "is likely." These are all perfectly acceptable terms, of course, but a single sentence that includes more than two hedges is not cogent.

Let's fix our earlier examples.

Example #1: *Alternatively, and in our view, far more likely, it is possible that if edema forms during the obstruction, it may be roentgenologically masked, perhaps by increases in lung volume.*

Removing all but one hedge leaves us with:

Alternatively, if edema forms during the obstruction it may be roentgenologically masked by increases in lung volume.

"Perhaps" could be retained as a second hedge, but six is far too many.

Example #2: *It is possible that some infections may take place among some patients in particular circumstances spontaneously*

We can rewrite this as:

Some infections may take place among patients spontaneously.

I have retained one hedge, and the considerable uncertainty in the original sentence has been brought under control.

Example #3: *Our study suggests that the beneficial effects of FMT may not be mediated solely through improvement in glycemic response.*

We can rewrite this as:

The beneficial effects of FMT may not be mediated solely through improvements in glycemic response.

I hope you get the idea by now: Avoid hedging whenever and wherever you can!

Professor Strunk also advises us to use the active, as opposed to the passive, voice, whenever possible. This advice is given often in English classes from middle school to university. In scientific prose, the passive voice is sometimes appropriate or even expected, but, in general, using the active voice as often as possible is more powerful and more cogent.

For example:

The first case of epilepsy I ever encountered will always be remembered.

Rewrite this as:

I will always remember the first case of epilepsy I encountered.

To convince yourself that the rewrite using the active voice is more cogent, imagine that the sentence is the beginning of a touching piece about a young boy diagnosed with epilepsy. Which version do you think would be more persuasive in getting you to read further?

Here's an example from the diabetes search:

Exercise is generally recommended for people with type 2 diabetes.

This can be rewritten using the active voice as:

Guidelines generally recommend exercise for individuals with type 2 diabetes.

As I noted, the passive voice is sometimes perfectly fine, or even preferred according to the style conventions of specific journals. That having been said, when permissible, please avoid it. If you want to make your writing more cogent, use the word "we" often. I say "we" since few scientific papers, abstracts, or grant applications are put together by one individual.

For example:

The patients were recruited from three health centers in Sacramento.

becomes

We recruited the patients from three health centers in Sacramento.
*   The participants were supported by the research team when adverse events occurred.*

becomes

We supported the participants when they experienced adverse events.

If you've already completed a work of scientific prose, go through it carefully to find places where you could have used the active voice instead of the passive voice.

Professor Strunk offers one last rule I place in the "cogency" category. Fortunately, it's relatively easy to follow. To make your writing more cogent, "put statements in positive form." Sometimes failing to do so can make a sentence very confusing. Consider this example from a paper:

Depression is no longer not considered to be a criterion for exclusion from participation in the program.

I had to read that sentence three times to understand it correctly. There are three negatives: "no longer," "not considered," and "exclusion." Unless you read the sentence carefully (likely at least twice), it's hard to know if participants with depression can participate in the program or not. If we put the statement in positive, it reads:

Depression is once again a criterion for exclusion from participation in the program.

Here's an example from the diabetes search:

Since HbA1c is measured once every 3 months and does not reflect the change in blood glucose promptly, HbA1c was not appropriate for assessing glycemic control in patients with adjusted hypoglycemic agents for less than 3 months.

A simple change from "was not appropriate" to "inappropriate" puts the main idea of the sentence in positive form:

Since HbA1c is measured once every 3 months and does not reflect the change in blood glucose promptly, HbA1c was inappropriate for assessing glycemic control in patients with adjusted hypoglycemic agents for less than 3 months.

"Inappropriate" is more powerful and convincing than "was not appropriate." Imagine you are at a party and are told a guest's behavior was "inappropriate." It sure sounds worse than if his behavior "was not appropriate."

My best advice to you is to keep this rule in mind as you write, and to review your writing once completed for statements that can be converted from negative to positive form to make them more cogent.

Commonness

The next "C" is the foundation of advice not only from Professor Strunk, who advises us to "avoid fancy words," but from many other writers, editors, and experts. I use "commonness" to refer to the use of the simplest or most common word whenever possible. In my experience, this is an especially significant challenge for biomedical writers. Granted, you can't avoid using jargon specific to the subject of a particular manuscript—"glucagon-like-peptide 1 agonist" is an example of an unavoidable term in a contemporary paper about diabetes. But using lots of flowery, unnecessary jargon makes it harder for readers to understand your message. Consider also that the audience for many journals, abstracts, books, etc. is international. Using fancy English words compromises your ability to be understood by many.

Here is an example I've used in many writing workshops:

Years in the trenches of primary care have, to some extent, inured me to biomedical failure if not to patients' suffering, so that the frustrations of my three unhurried consultations were not as poignant as they once might have been.

The passage is from an editorial piece, so you could argue that poetic license permits the author to use "fancy words" at his discretion. It's possible the author chose those words over others because they sounded more poetic, sophisticated, or elegant:•

- *Trenches of primary care*—Too many people in difficult occupations describe themselves as being "in the trenches."
- *Inured*—This word, neither commonly used nor easily understood, means hardened or grown accustomed to.
- *Biomedical failure*—I am at a loss for what this precisely means, and I'm both a physician and a scientist. I suppose it means an unfortunate or poor outcome.
- *Unhurried consultations*? If these were relaxed primary care visits, then the authors should state that plainly.
- *Poignant*? I've asked groups of highly educated workshop attendees to define poignant, and surprisingly few know that it means evoking sadness or regret. I wonder if that's what the author actually meant to say. He uses *frustrations* prior to poignant, and I believe that's enough to capture the intended meaning.

Writers should avoid pompous writing, as described in the introductory chapter. I read the sentence above a few times and interpreted is as follows:

Through my years in primary care, I've grown accustomed to poor outcomes if not to patients' suffering, so that my three relaxed patient visits weren't as frustrating as they once might have been.

The original sentence is a notable violation of the advice to "avoid fancy words" and isn't typical of what we might find in a scientific article. But many unnecessarily fancy words and jargon appear repeatedly in scientific papers. Although they've almost become standardized expressions, they can be trimmed or simplified to make the writing more accessible or "common" to all.

Let's return to our diabetes article search:

SGLT2 inhibitors have emerged as powerful agents to reduce the incidence of renal events, as well as cardiovascular events, in patients with type 2 diabetes.

It's not a bad sentence overall, but it could be revised in several ways—shortened or reorganized. The unnecessary "fanciness" is the term "have emerged," which has been used countless times in many pieces I've read. What does it really mean if a class of drugs has emerged, anyway? I would rewrite the sentence as:

In patients with type 2 diabetes, SGLT2 inhibitors reduce renal and cardiovascular events.

I suppose I could have retained "powerful agents," but I wonder if it really adds much given that the entire paper is about SGLT2 agents, and their power would have become apparent elsewhere in it.

So how does one go about keeping language simple?

1. Remember that using fancy words doesn't make your writing smart; in fact, they have quite the opposite effect. Knowing that should help.
2. As you write, keep each sentence as short and simple as possible. Simple words are usually shorter, so conciseness and commonness can work together to simplify your writing.
3. There are certain expressions that appear over and over again that add unnecessary pomposity to scientific writing. In addition to the list of Dreyer's "trimmables" in Table 2.1, Table 2.2 lists a few more and how I would handle them. As an exercise, go through a page in any published manuscript and find at least two "trimmables."
4. Imagine that you are writing for an educated person who has an interest in and knowledge of the subject of your paper (e.g., a fellow scientist) but whose mother tongue is not English. Apart from the necessary technical jargon, you'll want to choose the simplest words possible.

Consistency

Consistency is the simplest and perhaps most obvious of the 5Cs and is aligned with Professor Strunk's advice to "use a suitable design." Consistency

Table 2.2 More Phrases to Shorten

In terms of → about
The fact that → since (or just leave out if you can)
In order to → to
First and foremost → First, or firstly
In the event that → If

refers to writing in a way that is consistent with the expectations of the bio-medical reader. Indeed, the remainder of this book is all about consistency. Scientific writing is inherently complex, and adding structure to it helps us absorb information correctly, efficiently, and in the order the author intended. Following the appropriate design or form for scientific writing is essential. Experienced readers of the biomedical literature are so accustomed to the conventional structures of scientific writing, whether in the form of papers, grants, abstracts, or other forms, that deviations from the accepted form become immediately noticeable and sometimes infuriating. I serve on a study section for a federal grants review committee. When some part of a grant application is not in the expected place (or is absent) or else is not written in a form the review committee is accustomed to, the reaction is immediately harsh, even if the ideas in the application are sound. My advice to you is to familiarize yourself with the "suitable designs" of the most common biomedical writing tasks (i.e., those described in the following chapters).

Here is a clear published example of "violating the rules" (not from the diabetes search) that those of you who are clinicians like me might especially appreciate:

> *Mr. H, a sixty-six-year-old man, presented with retrosternal chest pain of two hours' duration. He reported no associated dizziness, dyspnea, or jaw pain. He has no allergies. He smokes roughly 1 pack of cigarettes per day. The pain was in his upper chest, and according to him felt like "someone sitting on his chest." His brother suffered a myocardial infarction last year. Mr. H takes amlodipine for hypertension, but no other medications. He was in mild respiratory distress with a modestly elevated respiratory rate. He looked pale, and was slightly agitated. He reported that he had not had symptoms of this type before and had good exercise tolerance prior to today.*

What's wrong with this case presentation is fairly obvious: The description mixes information from the patient's history with physical exam findings, with his smoking habits and allergies thrown into the mix as well. Almost all clinicians religiously follow a logical order in case presentations, in oral presentations of cases, and in documentation in the patient's medical record—history followed by physical examination. Habits such as smoking, drinking alcohol, along with allergies, family history etc. are usually described in distinct sections as well. I offer you this example not because violations of this type are common, but because I found it immediately irksome and a bit hard to follow. The same attention to consistency applies to all common forms of biomedical writing, to which we'll turn our attention in the chapters that follow.

5Cs Exercises and Suggested Responses

Exercise 1

Split the 71-word-sentence below into four shorter sentences to make it easier to digest. You may add a few words that help tie each sentence to the one that precedes it.

Effective management of diabetes involves a comprehensive approach that encompasses lifestyle modifications, including dietary changes, regular physical activity, and weight management, in addition to pharmacological interventions such as insulin therapy or oral medications, all of which must be tailored to the individual's specific needs and preferences, while also addressing comorbidities and minimizing the risk of complications through vigilant monitoring of blood glucose levels, periodic health assessments, and education about self-care practices.

Suggested response:

Managing diabetes effectively involves a comprehensive approach encompassing lifestyle modifications including dietary changes, regular physical activity, and weight management. Pharmacological interventions such as insulin therapy or oral medications are also important. All interventions must be tailored to the individual's specific needs. Effective management also involves addressing comorbidities while minimizing the risk of complications through vigilant monitoring of blood glucose levels, periodic health assessments, and education about self-care practices.

Exercise 2

Fix the following sentences with dangling, misplaced, or squinting modifiers.

Example 1

Having struggled with obesity for years, the new diet plan seemed promising.

Suggested response:

Having struggled with obesity for years, she thought the new diet plan seemed promising.

Example 2

While attempting to exercise regularly, the gym's crowded atmosphere often discouraged her.

Suggested response:

Although she attempted to exercise regularly, the gym's crowded atmosphere often discouraged her.

Example 3

Despite his reluctance, the doctor recommended pulmonary rehabilitation for the patient.

Suggested response:

The doctor recommended pulmonary rehabilitation for the patient, despite the patient's reluctance.

Example 4

Inhaling the bronchodilator rapidly reduces wheezing.

Suggested response:

Inhaling the bronchodilator reduces wheezing rapidly.

Exercise 3

Identify the hedges in this passage. Remove all but one (your choice).

The recent meta-analysis suggests that there may be a potential association between certain components of air pollution and possible cardiovascular outcomes, though we propose a cautious approach to drawing conclusions about the magnitude of the association.

The hedges here include "meta-analysis suggests," "there may be," "a potential association," "possible cardiovascular outcomes," and "we propose a cautious approach." A relatively hedge-free rewrite that carries largely the same meaning is:

The recent meta-analysis identifies an association between certain components of air pollution and cardiovascular outcomes, but the magnitude of the association is uncertain.

Exercise 4

This sentence below is 74 words long. Shorten it by at least half while retaining largely the same meaning:

The presence of elevated levels of circulating free fatty acids in the bloodstream has been implicated in the pathogenesis of various metabolic disorders such as obesity, insulin resistance, type 2 diabetes mellitus, and cardiovascular diseases, through adverse metabolic effects including impaired insulin signaling, increased hepatic gluconeogenesis, enhanced lipotoxicity, and heightened inflammatory responses, thus highlighting the importance of targeting free fatty acid metabolism as a potential therapeutic strategy for mitigating the progression of these conditions.

Suggested response:

Through adverse effects on insulin signaling, hepatic gluconeogenesis, lipotoxicity, and inflammation, free fatty acids are implicated in obesity, insulin resistance, type 2 diabetes, and cardiovascular diseases and are therefore an important therapeutic target. (33 words)

Exercise 5

What's wrong with this paragraph from the methods section of a health services research paper on heart failure?

Using an established computable phenotype, we queried our electronic data warehouse to identify patients with established heart failure with a minimum of two hospitalizations in 2024, who had been discharged to the remote monitoring program. Among the sixty-three identified patients, forty-one agreed to be interviewed about their experience.

While perfectly easy to understand, if the paragraph is from the methods section, it should include only methods. The number of patients identified through the query and the number who agreed to be interviewed are actually results and should be included in that section. This is a common problem we'll discuss later on in the book.

3
Writing a Paper

The Introduction

With some minor variations that apply to different sorts of papers, there are four basic elements of a biomedical paper: the introduction, methods, results, and discussion (summarized with the familiar IMRAD acronym). Often, a separate short "conclusion" is added after the discussion. We'll go through each of the four main elements in detail, but first here are a few guiding principles as you make your way through these sections of the book:

1. There is no precise formula for writing a good scientific paper. How you write an introduction will be influenced heavily by a journal's instructions for authors, general conventions in any particular medical or biological discipline, space requirements, and other factors. Adopting one particular formula or format for the sections of a paper would be neither practical nor desirable since the end result may be far from reviewers', editors', or readers' expectations.

2. So if principle (1) is true, you might wonder: Why bother with learning how to write specific sections of a paper at all? One could find general requirements in a journal's instructions for authors and then proceed in a way that is original and independent but nevertheless aligned with a journal's expectations. I believe, however, that a basic standardized approach can be applied to most situations, and even where variations on this approach are called for, it provides a useful framework for you to organize what you wish to say in the most clear and efficient way possible. In other words, learning a basic approach will serve you well no matter what variations on that approach are needed or preferred.

3. The introduction is the gateway to the rest of the paper and can be considered a sales pitch for why the remaining content is important to read. It is an ideal task to which to apply the 5Cs, especially cogency and clarity. Be bold, with short, crisp, and even provocative sentences to draw your reader in. Too many convoluted introductions lose the reader's attention, making it a real chore to get through the rest of the paper.

4. The introduction is often written after other sections, which is natural, since its purpose is to establish the scope of your paper, and that scope needs to be fully fleshed out beforehand.

The following scenario is about writing an introduction for an original research paper and, like all my examples, comes from the broad domain of health services research and quality improvement. Introductions for other types of articles, such as review articles, might be slightly different, but the same general ideas apply.

Scenario: *There are significant racial disparities in hypertension control among older (age ≥ 60 years) patients. Oscar is a nephrologist and health disparities researcher who has designed, implemented, and evaluated a multifaceted intervention to improve control rates among older African Americans with hypertension in Cleveland, Ohio. The intervention is unique because it is led by pharmacists. Each time patients refill their antihypertensive medications, their home blood pressure values are reviewed, lifestyle education and advice on improving medication adherence is provided, and adjustments are made to therapy. Compared to a control intervention, Oscar's IHCOA (Improving Hypertension Control Among Older African Americans) intervention achieved a control rate that was 60% higher. He and his team have analyzed all the data and have prepared methods, results, and discussion sections for a manuscript to be submitted to a prestigious journal. He just needs a short abstract and introduction.*

Sound guidance on how to write a good introduction has been available for many years in papers and books, often as part of broader advice on how to write scientific papers. The target audience and specific content is highly variable—from advice on grammar and tense intended especially for those whose first language is not English[1] to discussions of models or frameworks for introductions borrowed from sources not specific to biomedical papers.[2] Some advice uses jargon such as "establishing a territory,"[3] which I don't think is necessary for our purpose. From the standpoint of basic principles, advice from currently available sources is consistent.

---

[1] Gray JA. Introduction sections: Where are we going and why should I care? AME Med J 2018;3:112.

[2] Nundy S, Kakar A, Bhutta ZA. How to write the introduction to a scientific paper. In: *How to practice academic medicine and publish from developing countries?* Springer, 2021:193–199. https://doi.org/10.1007/978-981-16-5248-6_17, accessed February 24, 2024.

[3] Nundy S, Kakar A, Bhutta ZA. How to write the introduction to a scientific paper. In: *How to practice academic medicine and publish from developing countries?* Springer, 2021:193–199. https://doi.org/10.1007/978-981-16-5248-6_17, accessed February 24, 2024.

First, the introduction is of paramount importance, as noted above, since it not only sets the stage for the rest of the paper but also has the added purpose of captivating the interest of readers so they are motivated to continue reading. Second, the introduction has often been described as an inverted funnel.[4] The broad top includes very general information, and the narrow bottom is the end of the introduction and includes one or more very specific statements. What drives the reader forward in the introduction is the *motivation* for the research. The reader must understand that the research addresses an important problem that has not been previously addressed.

There are recommendations for the length or number of paragraphs for an introduction, but I'm averse to rigid, formulaic approaches. Instead, keep a few essential elements in mind: The introduction should include what is known about a problem, what is unknown, and what research is to be described in the paper to address what is unknown. As you think about how to write an introduction, I recommend starting with putting down four short sentences without much detail, upon which you can build a complete introduction or else use as a framework. Here are four sentences Oscar might use as a framework:

1. Older African Americans with hypertension are less likely to achieve blood pressure control than other Americans.
2. A number of multifaceted interventions to address this disparity in blood pressure control have been developed but have had limited success.
3. Pharmacists, since they have regular contact with patients with hypertension, can play a pivotal role in helping patients achieve control, but the effectiveness of pharmacist-led interventions among patients with lower levels of control is unknown.
4. We sought to compare the effectiveness of a pharmacist-led intervention to a usual care intervention among older African Americans with hypertension.

Notice the direction of the sentences from general to specific and inclusion of what is known, what is unknown, and what has been done. Notice also that motivation drives the order of sentences from describing a serious problem to a gap in knowledge that ought to be addressed to how the gap was filled. I highly recommend you start with a four-piece framework like that above as

---

[4] Gray JA. Introduction sections: Where are we going and why should I care? AME Med J 2018;3:112.

you prepare your introduction. You can even use simple phrases rather than full sentences with even less detail, such as the following:

1. Control poor African Americans
2. Current multifaceted interventions suboptimal
3. Pharmacists' potential unknown
4. Compare pharmacist to usual care

As a next step I recommend that you fill in the framework with additional detail. Details should be accompanied by citations that substantiate each statement. Oscar's framework begins with the racial disparity in hypertension control. Let's add detail to accompany his first sentence:

Older African Americans with hypertension are less likely to achieve blood pressure control than other Americans. Muntner et al. report that even after adjusting for socioeconomic status and access to health care, older African Americans are 12% less likely to achieve blood pressure control than their white counterparts.[5]

For the sake of simplicity, I've included only one citation. Oscar may wish to add additional sentences to substantiate his opening sentences, but there is generally no need to overdo it. One or two sentences accompanied by citations is enough to make the point.

Oscar's second point describes multifaceted interventions and their limited success. This point should also be substantiated with a citation. His original initial sentence can also be expanded:

A number of multifaceted interventions that include patient education and feedback, provider feedback, reminders and educational interventions, and technology-intensive strategies have been developed to address blood pressure control. Unfortunately, most interventions have had little impact on racial disparities in control.[6]

Again, this example has been simplified greatly since we're focused on the writing, not the clinical content. There are actually examples of narrowing of racial disparities in hypertension control through intensification of

[5] Muntner P, Hardy ST, Fine LJ, et al. Trends in blood pressure control among US adults with hypertension, 1999–2000 to 2017–2018. JAMA 2020;324(12):1190–1200. doi:10.1001/jama.2020.14545
[6] Kressin NR, Long JA, Glickman ME, et al. A brief, multifaceted, generic intervention to improve blood pressure control and reduce disparities had little effect. Ethn Dis 2016 Jan 21;26(1):27–36. doi:10.18865/ed.26.1.27. PMID: 26843793; PMCID: PMC4738852.

treatment.[7] Also, Oscar may wish to provide more detail to substantiate his statement about lack of impact on disparities with one or two specific examples. But let's move on.

Oscar's next point is about what is unknown—the impact of pharmacist-led management. He might expand upon his third point in the following way:

Patients with hypertension have regular contact with pharmacists, who can therefore play an important role in helping patients achieve blood pressure control. A systematic review published in 2020 concluded that pharmacist-led interventions can be effective in achieving control of cardiovascular risk factors, including hypertension.[8]

Next, Oscar can pivot to what is specifically unknown:

However, it is unknown if pharmacist-led interventions are effective in achieving control among older African Americans with hypertension compared with usual care.

Describing the gap in knowledge should make the motivation for Oscar's study obvious. He can expand upon his last point in the following way:

Our goal was to compare a multifaceted pharmacist-led intervention designed for older African Americans with hypertension to usual clinical care for achieving blood pressure control.

The statements above are sufficient for an introduction. Adding additional detail and examples is reasonable. It's also reasonable to include some aspects of the methods, such as "*Our goal was to compare, in a randomized trial, a multifaceted . . .*" Too much detail about methods is inappropriate since we have a whole other section in which to describe them. Let's put Oscar's draft introduction together:

Older African Americans with hypertension are less likely to achieve blood pressure control than other Americans. Muntner et al. report that even after adjusting for socioeconomic status and access to health care, older African

[7] Still CH, Rodriguez CJ, Wright JT Jr, et al. Clinical outcomes by race and ethnicity in the Systolic Blood Pressure Intervention Trial (SPRINT): A randomized clinical trial. Am J Hypertens 2017 Dec 8;31(1):97–107. doi:10.1093/ajh/hpx138. PMID: 28985268; PMCID: PMC5861531

[8] Alshehri AA, Jalal Z, Cheema E, et al. Impact of the pharmacist-led intervention on the control of medical cardiovascular risk factors for the primary prevention of cardiovascular disease in general practice: A systematic review and meta-analysis of randomised controlled trials. Br J Clin Pharmacol 2020 Jan;86(1):29–38. doi:10.1111/bcp.14164. Epub 2020 Jan 3. PMID: 31777082; PMCID: PMC6983518.

Americans are 12% less likely to achieve blood pressure control than their white counterparts.[9] A number of multifaceted interventions that include patient education and feedback, provider feedback, reminders and educational interventions, and technology-intensive strategies have been developed to address blood pressure control. Unfortunately, most interventions have had little impact on racial disparities in control.[10] Patients with hypertension have regular contact with pharmacists, who can therefore play an important role in helping patients achieve blood pressure control. A systematic review published in 2020 concluded that pharmacist-led interventions can be effective in achieving control of cardiovascular risk factors, including hypertension.[11] However, it is unknown if pharmacist-led interventions are more effective among older African Americans with hypertension compared with usual care.

The introduction is a single paragraph. Depending upon space limitations, Oscar could also write four separate paragraphs, each with additional detail. Oscar's introduction is perfectly reasonable in several ways. It moves in a logical direction, making the motivation for his study clear. It uses sentences of appropriate length, avoids jargon, and is generally clear and concise. But is it cogent? Does it grab your attention, or does it seem dry and generic? The next step may be unnecessary, but I would advise you to consider adding some boldness or "oomph" to your scientific writing. If the introduction is the entryway or sales pitch to the rest of the article, it should stand out and captivate the reader. There is no right or wrong way to do this. Always keep the basic rules of cogency in mind (active voice, statements in positive form, avoid hedging). Oscar hasn't violated any of these rules, so making his introduction more cogent requires a different approach. Consider this revision:

Hypertension has a terrible impact on the health and well-being of older Americans in the form of stroke, heart disease, and other complications. Older African Americans are especially affected by these problems, and it's truly unfortunate that they are less likely to achieve blood pressure control than other groups.[12] Multifaceted interventions that include patient and provider

[9] Muntner P, Hardy ST, Fine LJ, et al. Trends in blood pressure control among US adults with hypertension, 1999–2000 to 2017–2018. JAMA 2020;324(12):1190–1200. doi:10.1001/jama.2020.14545

[10] Kressin NR, Long JA, Glickman ME, et al. A brief, multifaceted, generic intervention to improve blood pressure control and reduce disparities had little effect. Ethn Dis 2016 Jan 21;26(1):27–36. doi:10.18865/ed.26.1.27. PMID: 26843793; PMCID: PMC4738852.

[11] Alshehri AA, Jalal Z, Cheema E, et al. Impact of the pharmacist-led intervention on the control of medical cardiovascular risk factors for the primary prevention of cardiovascular disease in general practice: A systematic review and meta-analysis of randomised controlled trials. Br J Clin Pharmacol 2020 Jan;86(1):29–38. doi:10.1111/bcp.14164. Epub 2020 Jan 3. PMID: 31777082; PMCID: PMC6983518.

[12] Muntner P, Hardy ST, Fine LJ, et al. Trends in blood pressure control among US adults with hypertension, 1999–2000 to 2017–2018. JAMA 2020;324(12):1190–1200. doi:10.1001/jama.2020.14545

Table 3.1 The 5Cs and the Introduction of a Paper

Conciseness	Introductions should be concise and serve the purpose of describing the motivation for the paper. Avoid too much supporting information and information that belongs elsewhere, such as details of the methods.
Cogency	In addition to the basics of avoiding hedging, putting statements in positive form, and using the active voice, be bold. Use short sentences with a powerful, unambiguous message.
Clarity	Clarity applies to an introduction as it does to any other form of scientific writing.
Commonness	An introduction is an especially important place to avoid jargon. Unfamiliar terms, if needed, should be defined.
Consistency	Move in a logical direction from the general to the highly specific and from describing the problem (what is known), to what is unknown, and to how the described research addresses what is unknown. Always end with a clear statement about the motivation for the research.

education, feedback, phone apps, etc., have been developed to improve control, but, sadly, their impact on older African Americans has been limited.[13] *What about the potential role of pharmacists? They have plenty of contact with patients, for example, when they refill medications. Could they play a role in helping older African Americans achieve better blood pressure control? We simply don't know, and our purpose in this study was to find out, by comparing a pharmacist-led intervention to usual care.*

I wrote this introduction keeping in mind Oscar's basic framework but striving to make each sentence bold and designed to keep a reader's attention. I urge you to try to do the same thing after writing a basic introduction like Oscar's example. You might wonder if the way in which I've rewritten his introduction might be stylistically unacceptable to a scientific journal. That's possibly true, but I'm an editor myself and welcome more cogent introductions. As the likelihood of publication will be based more on your methods, your results, and the overall quality of your work, I don't believe there's any harm in trying to be bold with an introduction designed to excite both reviewers and readers.

Cogency makes introductions stand out. The other 5Cs apply to an introduction as they do to any other form of scientific writing. Nevertheless, Table 3.1 describes application of the 5Cs in more detail.

---

[13] Kressin NR, Long JA, Glickman ME, et al. A brief, multifaceted, generic intervention to improve blood pressure control and reduce disparities had little effect. Ethn Dis 2016;26(1):27–36. doi:10.18865/ ed.26.1.27

Introduction Exercise

Here's a sample introduction to a scientific paper about peer counseling for depression among seniors:

> *We compared a peer-counseling intervention (PEER) in combination with primary care management of depression to primary care management alone among seniors with major depression, since major depression was more common among seniors during the COVID-19 pandemic. Bartholomew et al. describe a significant impact of depression in combination with isolation resulting not only in typical vegetative symptoms of depression but also worse physical health overall and worse self-management of chronic disease during the pandemic. Peers have been used successfully to enhance the effect of depression treatment interventions among postpartum women and other groups through the use of virtual communication. Whether virtual peer counseling is effective for seniors, a population less tech-savvy than others, is unclear.*

Rewrite this introduction based on what you've learned in this chapter. There is clearly some key information missing from it. You may use only what's there or supplement it with information from other sources.

Suggested Response

This introduction is clearly a mess in several ways: It doesn't move logically from general to more specific information, and the motivation, while described, needs to be more emphatic at the end. The acronym for the peer-counseling intervention is PEER, which isn't spelled out. Only one reference is cited. Here's one way to rewrite the introduction (specific references not included):

> *Depression takes a significant toll on the well-being of senior citizens, in terms of mental health, physical health, and the ability of seniors to self-manage chronic disease. Depression was more common and impactful during the COVID-19 pandemic. It has been shown that supplementing primary care management of depression with counseling provided by peers through virtual (online) communication is more effective than primary care management alone for specific groups, such as women with postpartum depression. However, whether virtual peer counseling can also benefit senior citizens in*

the same way is unknown. Seniors are less tech-savvy than other groups, and this factor may influence the success of virtual peer counseling. Our goal was to compare a virtual peer-counseling intervention with primary care management to primary care management alone among senior citizens with major depression.

4

Writing the Methods Section of Your Paper

The methods section usually follows the introduction in a biomedical paper and is arguably the most important. Van Calster et al. point out that poor and incompletely described methods sections in papers were common during the height of the COVID-19 pandemic, during which the rush to respond quickly to the public health emergency allowed a great deal of questionable research to be published.[1] The problem of poor methodology and incompletely described methodology was recognized long before the pandemic, and a number of efforts, including the development of reporting tools (see below) to promote completeness and transparency, have been promoted. The scope of this chapter is limited: I want you to be able to write a clear and complete methods section that meets accepted standards and makes your manuscript more likely to be accepted for publication. While the soundness of your methods is of critical importance, this book is about writing, not about high methodological standards for research. That having been said, the numerous reporting guidelines for different types of papers will help you follow accepted methodology, since standards for reporting must by necessity reflect sound methods.

Also, just as with a paper's introduction, the standards for how to write a methods section can vary greatly depending upon the journal, discipline, and type of research being carried out. For instance, the approach to the methods section of a systematic review on self-management approaches to heart failure would be quite different than that to a randomized trial involving hormonal responses to a new drug in mice. Like the introduction, however, I believe keeping in mind a few basic principles while you write your methods section and following the basic examples in this book will help you write clear and complete methods sections. These principles are as follows:

[1] Van Calster B, Wynants L, Riley RD, et al. Methodology over metrics: Current scientific standards are a disservice to patients and society. J Clin Epidemiol 2021Oct;138:219–226. doi:10.1016/j.jclinepi.2021.05.018. Epub 2021 May 30. PMID: 34077797; PMCID: PMC8795888.

1. As you write your methods section, keep in mind its two-fold purpose: helping readers understand your study and determine if the methods are valid, and helping others with a similar level of expertise as you to replicate or build upon your work.[2] While the introduction is the "hook" for the paper, the methods are the "nuts and bolts" of what was done, and anyone who is seriously interested in your paper will pay very close attention to them.

2. Completeness of methods should guide how you write this section. In fact, while your writing should always follow the 5Cs and be both clear and concise, you need to include as much detail as possible about what was done, why, and how. If the length of your methods section is constrained by a journal's standards, it's frequently possible to include additional detail in a supplement, often posted online. In other words, while your sentences and paragraphs should be concise, don't leave anything out! The default strategy is to include as much about the methods as possible. Let a journal's reviewers and editor decide if a part of what you've included is unimportant. It's been suggested that the methods section should include enough detail for you to replicate your own work faithfully a few years after you've published your paper.[3]

3. Organize your methods section according to accepted categories such as patients or participants, description of interventions, outcomes measured, statistical analysis methods, and ethical approvals. The number and types of such categories will vary depending upon the type of article, the discipline, and a journal's recommendations.

4. Always adhere to recommended reporting guidelines for your type of article. More about this below.

5. Stick to what was done, how, and why, and don't include anything that resembles a result in your methods section. For example, for the systematic review mentioned above about self-management of heart failure, there may have been a final set of 10 papers included. You shouldn't include a line such as, "Each of the 10 papers was reviewed by authors AM and SD," since the inclusion of 10 papers through a search and critical appraisal process is a result, not a method.

6. Define or explain methods that may be unfamiliar to your readers. For example, you may have analyzed the results of a cluster randomized trial

---

[2] How to write your methods. https://plos.org/resource/how-to-write-your-methods/. Accessed March 9, 2024.

[3] How to write your methods. https://plos.org/resource/how-to-write-your-methods/. Accessed March 9, 2024.

using Bayesian hierarchical models. While you should undoubtedly include detailed information about how such models were applied, it would be best to begin your description with something like, "Bayesian hierarchical models are statistical models that incorporate prior information and are useful for accommodating complex data structures and missing data."

<u>Scenario</u>: *Fatima is a behavioral health researcher and public health advocate who designed and carried out a randomized trial comparing St. John's wort, a flowering plant used for many ailments including depression, to placebo for smoking cessation. She obtained funding for her study from a federal grant. The study protocol and all procedures have been carefully documented as required by the institutional review board (IRB) of her home institution. She wishes to document her methods carefully in a manuscript for submission to a highly reputable journal.*

This scenario involves a randomized controlled trial, and the format and approach to methods for other types of studies will be necessarily different. I recommend a stepwise approach to documentation of the methods, keeping the key principles above in mind.

Start by learning about what is expected in a description of methods. Consult widely accepted standards for reporting based on your type of study. The first stop should be the website of the EQUATOR network (Enhancing the Quality and Transparency of Health Research) (https://www.equator-network.org/). Fatima has completed a randomized trial. The most relevant reporting guideline is the CONSORT statement (Consolidated Standards of Reporting Trials).[4] CONSORT consists of 25 checklist items including those applicable to the methods section of a paper. There are many types of CONSORT statements including recommendations for herbal medicines, and even a recent set of recommendations for trials that involve artificial intelligence. Though St. John's wort could be considered an herbal or complementary or alternative medicine treatment, to keep things simple we'll consider the CONSORT statement in its basic form. Table 4.1 lists the 17 components CONSORT recommends for the methods section.[5]

---

[4] Schulz KF, Altman DG, Moher D; CONSORT Group. CONSORT 2010 statement: Updated guidelines for reporting parallel group randomized trials. Ann Intern Med 2010 Jun 1;152(11):726–732. doi:10.7326/0003-4819-152-11-201006010-00232. Epub 2010 Mar 24. PMID: 20335313.

[5] Schulz KF, Altman DG, Moher D; CONSORT Group. CONSORT 2010 statement: Updated guidelines for reporting parallel group randomized trials. Ann Intern Med 2010 Jun 1;152(11):726–732. doi:10.7326/0003-4819-152-11-201006010-00232. Epub 2010 Mar 24. PMID: 20335313.

Table 4.1 CONSORT Recommendations for Methods Sections

Trial design	3a	Description of trial design (such as parallel, factorial) including allocation ratio
	3b	Important changes to methods after trial commencement (such as eligibility criteria), with reasons
Participants	4a	Eligibility criteria for participants
	4b	Settings and locations where the data were collected
Interventions	5	The interventions for each group with sufficient details to allow replication, including how and when they were actually administered
Outcomes	6a	Completely defined pre-specified primary and secondary outcome measures, including how and when they were assessed
	6b	Any changes to trial outcomes after the trial commenced, with reasons
Sample size	7a	How was sample size determined?
	7b	When applicable, explanation of any interim analyses and stopping guidelines
Randomization		
Sequence generation	8a	The method used to generate the random allocation sequence
	8b	Type of randomization; details of any restriction (such as blocking and block size)
Allocation concealment mechanism	9	The mechanism used to implement the random allocation sequence (such as sequentially numbered containers), describing any steps taken to conceal the sequence until interventions were assigned
Implementation	10	Who generated the random allocation sequence, who enrolled participants, and who assigned participants to interventions
Blinding	11a	If done, who was blinded after assignment to interventions (e.g., participants, care providers, those assessing outcomes) and how
	11b	If relevant, description of the similarity of interventions
Statistical methods	12a	Statistical methods used to compare groups for primary and secondary outcomes
	12b	Methods for additional analyses, such as subgroup analyses and adjusted analyses

Notice the amount of detail recommended.

I recommend you follow reporting guidelines closely. Keep in mind that all this information should be readily available to you already in the grant application, study protocol, and clinical trial registration. Always keep in mind that it's better to say too much than too little. Extract the relevant methods checklist from the EQUATOR network and add a column for your description of each item. Some checklist items, however, may not be applicable.

However, 17 subheadings are too many for a methods section for most journals. I would recommend you consolidate the information from your methods table into a smaller number of categories. Many clinical trials papers published in the *Journal of the American Medical Association* (JAMA) have an elegant structure for this that divides methods into study design, participants, procedures, outcomes, sample size, and statistical analysis.[6] What's important is that you organize your methods in a logical manner. Beyond that, where you put each type of relevant information is less important than being comprehensive.

Here's Fatima's methods section, with notes highlighting key features:

Study Design: *The ST3 (St. John's Wort to Stop Tobacco Smoking in a Timely Fashion) was a placebo-controlled parallel-group double-blinded randomized trial of 52 weeks duration that took place in Pittsburgh, PA, between August 1, 2023, and June 30, 2025. The study protocol was approved by the University of Pittsburgh and followed the principles of the Declaration of Helsinki.*

It's reasonable to include ethical approvals here.

Participants: *Eligible participants were adult (age ≥ 18 years) daily cigarette smokers with a Cigarette Dependence (short version) Scale (CDS-5) score of 4.0 or higher.[7] Key exclusion criteria included simultaneous use of other nicotine products including electronic cigarettes and chewing tobacco, or being currently engaged in a quit attempt, including use of any smoking cessation product or medication, known allergy to St. John's wort, inability to read and understand English, and inability to travel to the research procedures and coordinating site at the University of Pittsburgh, where all data were collected.*

I recommended describing unfamiliar methods in detail. Fatima could have provided additional details about the Cigarette Dependence Scale. She has instead provided a citation, which is a perfectly reasonable alternative.

To organize information in lengthier parts of the methods section, such as the following description of procedures, in a way that is easier for readers to absorb, use as many section subheadings as you believe you need.

[6] Aronne LJ, Sattar N, Horn DB, et al.; SURMOUNT-4 Investigators. Continued treatment with tirzepatide for maintenance of weight reduction in adults with obesity: The SURMOUNT-4 randomized clinical trial. JAMA 2024 Jan 2;331(1):38–48. doi:10.1001/jama.2023.24945. PMID: 38078870; PMCID: PMC10714284.

[7] Etter JF, Le Houezec J, Perneger TV. A self-administered questionnaire to measure dependence on cigarettes: The Cigarette Dependence Scale. *Neuropsychopharmacology* 2003;28(2):359–370. doi:10.1038/sj.npp.1300030

Procedures

Recruitment of Participants: *Participants were recruited from primary care offices throughout the greater Pittsburgh area, where flyers were distributed. Primary care physicians and practice managers were informed about and given details about the study including the study protocol, and were also encouraged to refer patients they felt would be willing to participate and could benefit. When patients called a toll-free number, a research assistant confirmed basic eligibility, including administration of the CDS-5 over the phone. Eligible participants who remained interested were asked to come to the central coordinating site, where eligibility was confirmed and informed consent obtained.*

Baseline Assessment: *After informed consent was obtained, we collected demographic information including age, sex, gender, race/ethnicity, and tobacco use history. We also asked about any medical history of chronic illnesses including pulmonary and cardiovascular history, as well as current medications. Readiness to quit was measured using the Contemplation Ladder.*[8]

Interventions: *Block randomization using blocks of six was carried out using SPSS version 27 (IBM, Armonk, NY). For allocation concealment, opaque, sequentially numbered envelopes containing the treatment assignments were prepared by an independent statistician prior to the start of the trial. These envelopes were opened only after participants were recruited and their baseline data were collected, ensuring that neither the participants nor the researchers involved in the trial were aware of the treatment allocation until after the baseline assessment. Participants were randomly assigned to St. John's wort (*Hypericum perforatum*) in the form of 0.3% extract in capsules of 300 mg (Western Herbals, Minneapolis, MN) to be taken three times daily or placebo for a period of 12 weeks.*

Outcomes: *The primary outcome was being abstinent from tobacco for 7 or more days after 12 weeks of treatment. Secondary outcomes were abstinence at 3 months, 6 months, and 1 year. Abstinence was confirmed if participants reported no intake of tobacco and their urinary cotinine level was <100 ng/mL (ELISA test, Calbiotech Co., Spring Valley, CA).*

[8] Biener L, Abrams DB. The Contemplation Ladder: Validation of a measure of readiness to consider smoking cessation. Health Psychol 1991;10:3605.

Statistical Methods: *Fisher's exact test was used to compare abstinent rates at each of the outcome time points. Multiple regression analysis was carried out to identify the relationship of treatment assignment and baseline variables upon abstinence outcomes at each time point. All statistical analyses were completed using SPSS version 27 (IBM, Armonk, NY).*

Sample Size: *Assuming a 1:1 allocation ratio, a 12-week abstinence rate of 15% in the placebo group and 30% in the St. John's Wort group, and a type 1 error rate of 0.05 and 80% power to detect a difference of 15% or greater in abstinent rates, we estimated that 120 participants were needed in each group.*

Fatima's descriptions of her methods are brief but they include all the elements of the CONSORT checklist.

The content of this sample methods section is deliberately simple; in reality, one might use more sophisticated statistical methods, for example. The important thing is that you understand the importance of including the essential elements and organize the methods in a way that is easy to understand. Table 4.2 describes the application of the 5Cs to methods.

Table 4.2 5Cs and Methods

Conciseness	You might think that conciseness doesn't apply based on what I've told you about being comprehensive. Your sentences should be short and crisp as always. At least for a first draft, don't worry about making your methods section too long. Write down as much detail as possible, and then trim the section down to meet journal requirements for the methods section or for the entire paper. Always take advantage of the opportunity to include additional information about methods in a supplement.
Cogency	As always, use the active voice and put statements in positive form—for instance, "We estimated 120 participants were needed in each group" rather than "An estimate of 120 participants per group was made."
Clarity	Clarity applies to the methods section as it does to any other form of scientific writing. Clarity will be enhanced by providing as much detail as possible.
Commonness	Make sure any acronyms are spelled out when you first use them. If you anticipate that a method is unfamiliar to potential readers, don't hesitate to add a sentence or two to describe it.
Consistency	Consistency is especially applicable to the methods section. Always consult an applicable reporting checklist and organize your methods in a logical fashion by reviewing prior published papers in the journal to which you are submitting.

Methods Exercise

Here's an example of a methods section that is poorly organized and lacks clarity. It is also missing key information. Your task is reorganize and rewrite the content so that it is easier to understand. Don't worry too much about being concise. As you rewrite, think also about what information is missing, and make notes about what else you would like to know about the methods that were used. The exercise of reorganizing a poorly written methods section and identifying key missing information should help you write methods sections that are clear and comprehensive.

We randomized (double-blind) medically stable patients ≥18 years of age with CHF, EF > 40%, and BNP ≥ 150pg/dL to sacubitril/valsartan or placebo who had had a recent hospitalization for CHF. Exclusion criteria included patients with significant valvular disease, genetic hypertrophic cardiomyopathy, or amyloid heart disease. Sacubitril/valsartan (Sac/Val) was provided at a dose titrated to 160 mg twice daily. Patients had to be hemodynamically stable with no symptomatic hypotension. Additional exclusion criteria included pregnancy, known hepatic impairment, confirmed COVID-19 infection, and estimated life expectancy <6 months. Informed consent was obtained prior to randomization. Patients were recruited from outpatient hospital clinics in the greater Samsonburg area. Institutional review board approval was obtained from Samsonburg District Hospital. Patients with a known history of hypersensitivity to ARNIs or ARBs were excluded. Outcomes included heart failure hospitalizations over the course of 52 weeks and cardiovascular deaths. Secondary outcomes included incidence of symptomatic hypotension, hyperkalemia, angioedema, or worsening renal function, defined as an increase in serum creatinine of ≥0.5 mg/dL and worsening of the eGFR by at least 25%. All patients had to be English-speaking with no documented evidence of cognitive impairment. Patients ≥80 years of age were excluded. Randomization was at a ratio of 1:1 with concealed allocation. To detect a 25% reduction in rate of hospitalization for CHF with Sac/VAL compared to placebo over the course of the 52-week trial, we estimated that a sample size of 200 patients per each group was needed with 85% power. To account for dropouts, we set a target of recruiting a total of 500 patients. The trial complies with the Declaration of Helsinki. All statistical analyses were completed by a statistician using the latest version of R.

Suggested Response

I based the disorganized methods paragraph above on a superbly organized description of a randomized trial (PARAGLIDE-HF trial) to which you may wish to refer as an example of detailed and clear methods.[9] A decent way to re-organize the methods would be to follow the scheme for Fatima's study. Note that you may wish to spell out some acronyms, but this is likely not necessary, since these may have been spelled out in the introduction. Also, additional details should be included in an actual methods section suitable for a manuscript submission. I've kept things simple, but point out where more information would be expected.

Study Design: *This was a double-blind, placebo-controlled 52-week randomized trial of sacubitril/valsartan versus placebo. The protocol was approved by Samsonburg District Hospital. The trial complies with the Declaration of Helsinki.*

Study Procedures
Participants: *Eligible participants included medically stable English-speaking patients ≥18 years but <80 years of age with CHF, EF > 40%, and BNP ≥ 150 pg/dL to sacubitril/valsartan or placebo who had had a recent hospitalization for CHF. Exclusion criteria included significant valvular disease, genetic hypertrophic cardiomyopathy, amyloid heart disease, known hepatic impairment, pregnancy, confirmed COVID-19 infection, history of hypersensitivity to ARNIs or ARBs, cognitive impairment, and estimated life expectancy <6 months.*

Recruitment: *Patients were recruited from outpatient hospital clinics in the greater Samsonburg area. Informed consent was obtained prior to randomization.*

Ideally, much more information about recruitment information should be included—for instance, How were potentially eligible patients identified? What recruitment procedures were followed? How and who obtained informed consent? Over what timeframe did recruitment take place?

No information about baseline assessment was included in the sample methods paragraph. This part of the methods section should include

[9] Mentz RJ, Ward JH, Hernandez AF, et al. Rationale, design and baseline characteristics of the PARAGLIDE-HF trial: Sacubitril/valsartan vs valsartan in HFmrEF and HFpEF with a worsening heart failure event. J Card Fail 2023 Jun;29(6):922–930. doi:10.1016/j.cardfail.2023.02.001. Epub 2023 Feb 14.

information such as the demographics, cardiac function, and comorbid conditions of potential participants.

Interventions: *Randomization was at a ratio of 1:1 with concealed allocation.*

More information is needed here, including any block or stratified randomization and the methods for concealed allocation.

Patients were randomized to sacubitril/valsartan (Sac/Val) at a dose titrated to 160 mg twice daily or twice-daily placebo.

How the dose was titrated should be included here, including over what timeframe.

Outcomes: *The primary outcome was heart failure hospitalizations over the course of 52 weeks and cardiovascular deaths. Secondary outcomes included incidence of symptomatic hypotension hyperkalemia, angioedema, or worsening renal function defined as an increase in serum creatinine of ≥0.5 mg/dL and worsening of the eGFR by at least 25%.*

The methods section should clearly specify that the primary outcome was heart failure hospitalizations over the 52-week period.

Statistical Methods: *All statistical analyses were completed by a statistician using the latest version of R.*

Obviously, more information is needed about what statistical methods were used.

Sample Size: *To detect a 25% reduction in rate of hospitalization for CHF with Sac/VAL compared to placebo over the course of the 52-week trial, we estimated that a sample size of 200 patients per each group was needed with 85% power. To account for dropouts, we set a target of recruiting a total of 500 patients.*

It would be helpful to know how and why the 25% reduction in rate of hospitalization that is the basis for this calculation was determined.

5

Writing Your Results Section

While the methods section is arguably the most important, as it reflects the integrity and validity of a scientific paper, the results section is the one that gets the most attention from consumers of research, including news organizations.[1] As with research methods, the content and format of a results section will vary greatly depending upon the type of paper, the audience, the journal, and the authors' perspectives on what findings are most important. Nevertheless, there are important principles to keep in mind and follow:

1. *Organization is critically important.* Writing up your results section haphazardly without respect for organizational conventions results in a jumbled mess, which makes it difficult for readers to understand, if it even makes it to publication. The order of elements is critically important. A common order for many clinical research studies is the following: results of recruitment, sample characteristics, findings from the primary analyses, findings from the secondary analyses, and any additional findings, including unexpected ones.[2]

2. *Be transparent and honest at all times.* Medical research literature is replete with examples of research misconduct in the form of exaggerated, incomplete, or false results. Roughly 2% of scientists admit to falsifying data and 14% report having observed falsification of data by colleagues.[3] While dishonesty in reporting is a serious problem, there is also the problem of "spin" —defined as "the use of specific reporting strategies, from whatever motive to highlight that the experimental treatment is beneficial, despite a statistically nonsignificant difference for the primary outcome, or to distract the reader from statistically nonsignificant

[1] Elsevier Author Services. How to write the results section of a research paper. https://scientific-publishing.webshop.elsevier.com/manuscript-preparation/how-to-write-the-results-section-of-a-research-paper/. Accessed April 6, 2024.

[2] Kotz D, Cals JWL. Effective writing and publishing scientific papers, part V: Results. J Clin Epidemiol 2013;66:945.

[3] Fanelli D. How many scientists fabricate and falsify research? A systematic review and meta-analysis of survey data. PLoS One 2009 May 29;4(5):e5738. doi:10.1371/journal.pone.0005738. PMID: 19478950; PMCID: PMC2685008.

results."[4] An example of spin includes emphasizing secondary outcomes in a paper rather than primary outcomes. Khan et al. reviewed randomized trials with statistically nonsignificant results published in six leading journals, including the *New England Journal of Medicine, Lancet,* and the *Journal of the American Medical Association* (JAMA). They found spin in the main text of 67% of papers.[5] Make sure your results section is accurate and complete and objectively summarizes the outcomes you prioritized at the outset.

3. *Use reporting guidelines.* As with your methods section, prior to writing up your results section, you should visit the website of the EQUATOR network and review the reporting guideline relevant to your type of paper. Reporting guidelines can't overcome misconduct or spin in reporting results, but they will help you organize your results appropriately and avoid missing key information. Citing a specific reporting guideline in your paper also adds credibility.

4. *Don't interpret your results in the results section.* Interpretation of results belongs in the discussion section of your paper. This seems obvious, but it is easy to add an element of interpretation in your results. For example, consider the following sentence: "Surprisingly, in the control group, 38% reported no symptoms at the 6-month point." The adverb "surprisingly," while seemingly innocuous, is an interpretation of the finding it precedes and belongs in the discussion section, not the results. Let your reader absorb your results objectively first and save the interpretation for the discussion.

5. *Use figures and tables generously when results are numerous or complex.* We'll spend considerable time on figures and tables in this chapter. Figures and tables are an extremely useful way to summarize results. Readers gravitate to them. They will make their way into PowerPoint presentations. Journals sometimes have a maximum number of allowable figures and tables but will also often allow you to include more in a supplement. The old adage "a picture is worth a thousand words" is especially apt for your results section. There are important style conventions for figures and tables, which we'll touch upon.[6]

[4] Boutron I, Dutton S, Ravaud P, Altman DG. Reporting and interpretation of randomized controlled trials with statistically nonsignificant results for primary outcomes. JAMA 2010;303(20):2058–2064.

[5] Khan MS, Lateef N, Siddiqi TJ, et al. Level and prevalence of spin in published cardiovascular randomized clinical trial reports with statistically nonsignificant primary outcomes: A systematic review. JAMA Netw Open 2019 May 3;2(5):e192622. doi:10.1001/jamanetworkopen.2019.2622. PMID: 3105775; PMCID: PMC6503494.

[6] Christiansen SL, Iverson C, Flanagin A, et al. *AMA manual of style: A guide for authors and editors* (11th ed.). Oxford University Press, 2020.

Table 5.1 CONSORT Checklist Items for Results of Randomized Trials

Participant flow (a diagram is strongly recommended)	13a	For each group, the numbers of participants who were randomly assigned, received intended treatment, and were analyzed for the primary outcome
	13b	For each group, losses and exclusions after randomization, together with reasons
Recruitment	14a	Dates defining the periods of recruitment and follow-up
	14b	Why the trial ended or was stopped
Baseline data	15	A table showing baseline demographic and clinical characteristics for each group
Numbers analyzed	16	For each group, number of participants (denominator) included in each analysis and whether the analysis was by original assigned groups
Outcomes and estimation	17a	For each primary and secondary outcome, results for each group, and the estimated effect size and its precision (such as 95% confidence interval)
	17b	For binary outcomes, presentation of both absolute and relative effect sizes is recommended
Ancillary analyses	18	Results of any other analyses performed, including subgroup analyses and adjusted analyses, distinguishing prespecified from exploratory
Harms	19	All important harms or unintended effects in each group (for specific guidance see CONSORT for harms)

Let's extend the example of Fatima's study on St. John's wort for smoking cessation (see Chapter 4) to the results section. As with the methods section, a stepwise approach to summarizing methods is helpful. The first stop once again should be the website of the EQUATOR network, through which the CONSORT statement can be located. The relevant checklist items are shown in Table 5.1. Keep in mind always that there are a number of reporting guidelines available for studies other than randomized trials.

The checklist is informative for what should be included as well as how to organize the section. It's reasonable to start with the first two items on the checklist, participant flow and recruitment. A flowchart shows "the sequence of activities, processes, events, operations or organization of a complex procedure or an interrelated system of components and sometimes function as visual summaries of a study." Useful recommendations on how to construct a flowchart as well as an additional broad range of stylistic conventions can be found in the *AMA Manual of Style: A Guide for Authors and Editors.* While this manual isn't a universally accepted guide to style, it is comprehensive in scope and widely used by authors, editors, and journals. I suggest following its recommendations unless a journal recommends otherwise. The recommendations are highly specific. For example, in a flowchart, an oval indicates randomized allocation whereas a rectangle represents non-random allocation. A flowchart is an excellent way to summarize patient flow through a clinical trial. It is reasonable to summarize key results for patient flow in the text of the paper, to accompany the flowchart.

Based on her study, Fatima wrote the following:

316 patients were initially identified as eligible. 126 were found to be ineligible. Among these, 74 were engaged in a quit attempt, 18 used chewing tobacco only at the time of screening, 8 were not fluent in English, and 24 were ineligible as they did not meet the threshold of ≥ 4.0 on the CDS-5. 190 patients were randomized (98 to the St. John's wort group, and 92 to placebo). A total of 168 patients completed the trial. Trial flow is summarized in Figure 1.

This paragraph is intended to provide a quick, easy-to-read summary of participant flow through the study. The actual flow diagram can include additional details, including reasons for not completing the trial, and the number completing the trial in each group. Figure 5.1 shows Fatima's flow diagram, often labeled *Figure 1* in many descriptions of randomized trial results.

An appropriate next step would be to summarize characteristics of the sample of 168 patients. As with Figure 5.1, it's appropriate to include some information in the main text. More detailed information can be provided in a table, often titled *Table 1*. For a randomized trial, the sample is usually divided into intervention and control groups. In the past, differences in baseline characteristics between intervention and control groups were accompanied by p-values. P-values were often included to demonstrate the success of randomization. However, this practice is now considered misleading and is now actively discouraged.[7] In the table, it's reasonable to provide standard deviations (SDs) to accompany mean values, and percentages to accompany absolute counts.

Fatima's text for baseline characteristics is as follows:

A total of 122 women and 68 men were enrolled. The mean age of all participants was 51.3 years. The median CDS-5 score was 5.9 (SD, 1.2) in the St. John's wort group and 5.8 (SD, 1.6) in the placebo group. Participants in the intervention group smoked an average of 18 (SD, 5.2) cigarettes a day;

---

[7] de Boer MR, Waterlander WE, Kuijper LD, et al. Testing for baseline differences in randomized controlled trials: An unhealthy research behavior that is hard to eradicate. Int J Behav Nutr Phys Act 2015;12, Article 4. https://doi.org/10.1186/s12966-015-0162-z

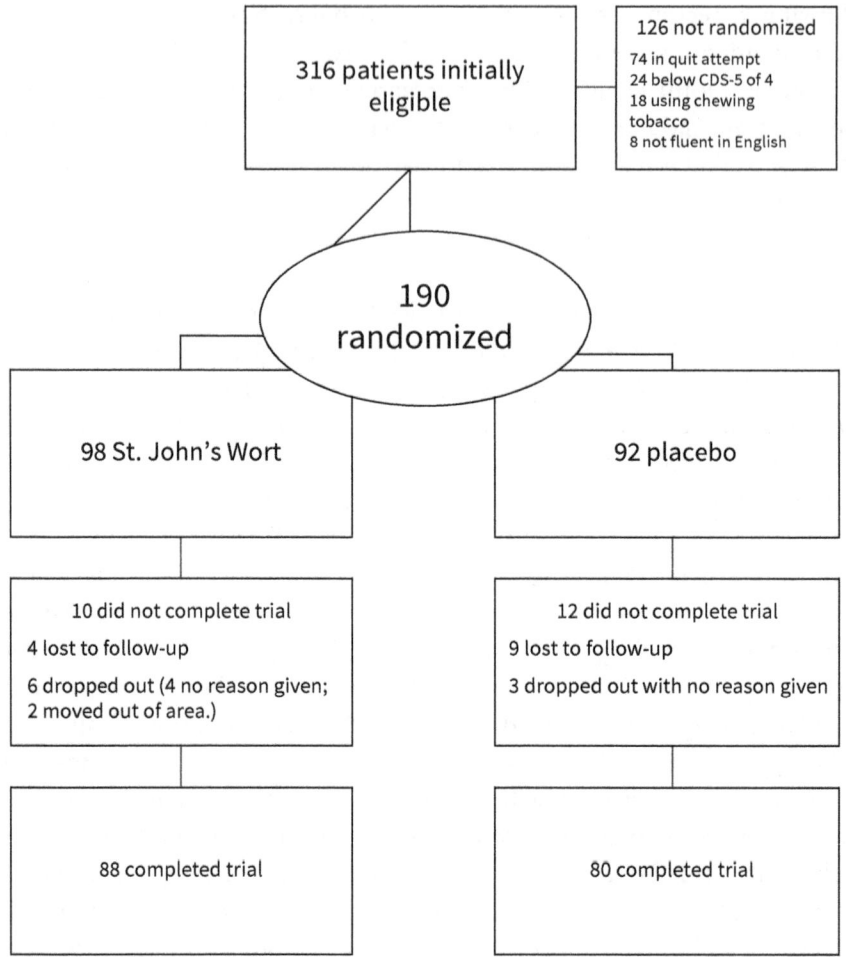

Figure 5.1 Flow of participants

those in the placebo group smoked an average of 16 (SD, 5.6) cigarettes a day. Additional baseline characteristics are summarized in Table 1.

Notice that the text provides some details to give readers an overview of the participants. However, not everything in the table should be summarized in paragraph form; that would be both unnecessary and difficult to read. The table, however, should be as detailed as possible. Table 5.2 shows Fatima's table for baseline characteristics.

Moving on to the general outline of results, the next section should be results from primary analyses. The primary outcome for Fatima's study is abstinence from tobacco for 7 or more days after 12 weeks of treatment. This

Table 5.2 Sample Baseline Characteristics of Participants Table

Characteristic	St. John's Wort (n = 98)	Placebo (n = 92)
Women (%)	64 (65)	58 (63)
Mean age (SD)	52.4 years (10.8)	50.8 (10.5)
Non-Hispanic White ancestry (%)	82 (84)	85 (92)
Married (%)	50 (51)	54 (59)
College graduate (%)	18 (18)	19 (21)
Mean cigarettes per day (SD)	18 (5.2)	16 (5.6)
Mean number of years smoked (SD)	31 (12.3)	26 (14.0)
One or more other smokers in household (%)	66 (67)	60 (65)
One or more previous quit attempts (%)	72 (73)	66 (72)
Mean CDS-5 score (SD)	5.9 (1.2)	5.8 (1.6)

important result can be summarized in a single sentence; there is no need for a table or figure. Sometimes a table is useful if the primary outcome has been analyzed further—for example, abstinence rates among men versus women, or another baseline characteristic, can be presented. Fatima's outcome, however, is quite simple, and even these primary outcomes by baseline characteristics can be summarized succinctly in text form. The primary outcome should include a measure of statistical significance.

Fatima's summary of the primary outcome is as follows:

Among 88 participants assigned to the St. John's wort group who completed the trial, 18 were abstinent at 12 weeks. Among 80 participants assigned to the placebo group who completed the trial, 15 were abstinent at 12 weeks. The p-value for the difference was 0.42. There were no significant differences in abstinence between the two groups based on baseline characteristics including sex, age (above or below mean), race/ethnicity, years of smoking, presence of one or more chronic illnesses, and Contemplation Ladder scores.

Fatima could have included numerical values with accompanying p-values for the abstinence rates in each group based on baseline characteristics or included these as a table. However, this is unnecessary, especially as she found no significant differences.

Fatima's secondary outcomes included abstinence at 3 months, 6 months, and 1 year. These can also be summarized in text form. Here is her summary:

At 3 months, 11 participants assigned to the St. John's wort group remained abstinent, compared to 6 in the placebo group (p < 0.05). At 6 months, 9 *participants assigned to the St. John's wort group remained abstinent, compared to 4 in the placebo group (p < 0.05). At 12 months, none of the participants in the trial were abstinent.*

This text summary is adequate for the secondary outcomes; once again, a table is unnecessary. An analysis by baseline characteristics is unnecessary, and may indeed be misleading, since the number of participants who remained abstinent at 3 and 6 months was so small. It may be tempting to begin the last sentence with "Unfortunately, at 12 months, none of the participants." However, "unfortunately" is an interpretation of the result that doesn't belong in the results section.

The final section of the summary of results can include additional findings, including unexpected ones. These should usually be linked to the methods. It's not appropriate, for example, to discuss side effects from the St. John's wort and placebo preparations if that wasn't one of the outcomes Fatima set out to measure. Fatima did uncover one unusual finding:

At 12 weeks, we found discrepancies between cotinine levels < 100 ng/mL and self-reported abstinence among 14 participants (9 in the St. John's wort group and 5 in the placebo group). These patients reported being abstinent but had cotinine levels above the threshold. As per our protocol, these patients were not considered to be abstinent.

Again, it's tempting to include some interpretation of this interesting result in the results section. Keep in mind, however, that even a simple qualifier such as "unusually," "strangely," or "unexpectedly" is an interpretation and belongs in the discussion section, not the results section.

I've provided this example of Fatima's study as a relatively simple one to illustrate some key principles. In reality, though, results from clinical trials may be considerably more complex and may include more tables and figures, but the same principles apply. Table 5.3 shows how the 5Cs are applicable to results section.

Results Exercise

Clinicaltrials.gov is an online database of clinical studies, intended for researchers and research consumers.[8] Results of clinical trials, when available,

---

[8] https://clinicaltrials.gov/about-site/about-ctg. Accessed April 15, 2024.

Table 5.3 Application of the 5Cs to Results

Conciseness	Key results should be included in text in short, sharp sentences that provide readers with highlights of the study they can easily absorb. Figures and tables are useful to summarize results when the equivalent text would be lengthy and cumbersome.
Cogency	Always put statements in positive form. However, the passive voice is often acceptable, depending upon a journal's stylistic conventions, when summarizing results (e.g., "346 patients were recruited" versus "We recruited 346 patients").
Clarity	Clarity is of course critical to all parts of a manuscript. The primary mechanism through which clarity is enhanced in the results section is through the use of figures and tables.
Commonness	Avoid jargon, as always. It's a good idea to spell out acronyms or provide definitions for complicated terms in the legends of figures and tables.
Consistency	Follow general reporting guidelines for the flow of the results section that is relevant to your study—for clinical trials, for example, patient flow, baseline characteristics, results from primary analyses, results from secondary analyses, and unexpected results.

are posted in a simple raw form, even before they are published as part of a paper. Your exercise is to review the clinicaltrials.gov posting for one specific trial with relatively simple results (https://www.clinicaltrials.gov/study/ NCT05049616) and to construct a results section based on the principles and recommendations in this chapter.

Suggested Response

Start by clicking on the "Results Posted" tab on the linked page above. This is a relatively small and simple trial. Details about how screening and recruitment were carried out are not provided. Three simple sentences about recruitment/ flow and randomization are appropriate.

> *A total of 70 women with postpartum hypertension were recruited. 34 participants were randomized to the HCTZ/lisinopril arm, and 36 to the extended-release nifedipine arm. Three patients in the HCTZ/lisinopril arm did not complete the study.*

An appropriate next component of the results section is a summary of baseline characteristics. You'll notice a large number of these, but some of them are not relevant. For example, all patients were recruited from the United States, so a breakdown of region for participants isn't needed. Some of these would be superfluous when submitting to a journal. For example, both the mean body mass index (BMI) and proportion of participants in each arm with a BMI $\geq$ 30 kg/m^2 (i.e., obesity) are given, but one measure of weight is sufficient. In some cases, the clinical details may be of lesser or greater importance. For example, the number of women in each group who underwent cesarean delivery may not be needed in your results section; you could include this and other clinical details in a supplemental table. Start your baseline characteristics summary with a short paragraph with a few key features of the entire sample. With characteristics that are dichotomous, you only need to mention one of the two categories in your summary paragraph.

Among the 67 women who completed the study, 23 (34.3%) were age 35 years or older. The majority, 40 (59.7%), were African American. Forty-five (67.2%) had obesity. Twenty-nine (43.3%) had chronic hypertension. Remaining characteristics of the overall sample and breakdown by treatment arm are shown in Table 1.

You may choose to insert more detail in your paragraph, including a breakdown of the age, race, obesity, and chronic hypertension characteristics by treatment arm. The key is to keep it short, since you'll provide this detail again in the table.

The table itself need not include everything you find on the clinicaltrials. gov page because this information will remain on the page after the paper is published. Instead, include key baseline characteristics for each group that are generally most relevant to a study about postpartum hypertension. A table that is too lengthy or complex will be difficult to absorb. Table 5.4 shows an example of an appropriate baseline characteristics table.

This table provides a useful general overview of the sample. You could choose to add additional available baseline characteristics or totals for the entire sample, but these are not necessary.

The next component of the results section should be your findings from the primary analyses. The first outcome listed according to the clinicaltrials. gov record is stage 2 hypertension on days 7 to 10 after delivery or admission to hospital for blood pressure control on or before day 10. It's reasonable to consider this to be one of the primary outcomes, along with severe postpartum hypertension. These two outcomes could be summarized in text form in a couple of sentences. Note that the CONSORT checklist recommends a measure of the effect size and a measure of precision such as 95% confidence intervals (CIs). Details of the statistical analysis methods of the data are not provided, and it's difficult to know what methods have been or will be applied.

Table 5.4 Sample Baseline Characteristics Table

		HCTZ/Lisinopril (n = 31)	Extended-Release Nifedipine (n = 36)
Age ≥ 35 years	Age ≥ 35 years	7 (22.6%)	16 (44.4%)
Race/ethnicity	Non-Hispanic Black	16 (51.6%)	24 (66.7%)
	Hispanic	9 (29.0%)	7 (19.4%)
	Non-Hispanic White	3 (9.7%)	4 (11.1%)
	Asian	3 (9.7%)	1 (2.8%)
Nulliparous		4 (12.9%)	7 (10.4%)
Obesity		20 (64.5%)	25 (69.4%)
Diabetes prior to pregnancy		6 (19.4%)	7 (19.4%)
Gestational diabetes		2 (6.5%)	5 (13.9%)
Chronic hypertension		14 (45.2%)	15 (41.7%)
Antihypertensive medication use in pregnancy		15 (48.4%)	13 (36.1%)
Hypertensive disorder during pregnancy		28 (90.3%)	31 (86.1%)
Needed IV BP medication prior to randomization		11 (35.5%)	11 (30.6%)

If you're interested, a common way to summarize the data is with odds ratios (ORs). You can calculate 95% CIs for ORs online (https://www.medcalc.org/calc/odds_ratio.php). However, this book is about writing, not biostatistics (I've written another book[9] that is largely about biostatistics in case you're interested!), so just note that you should include a measure of effect size and precision:

8/30 patients analyzed in the HCTZ/lisinopril group had stage 2 hypertension or needed antihypertensive treatment 7 to 10 days after delivery versus 12/28 patients in the extended-release nifedipine group (OR 0.48, 95% CI (0.16, 1.46)). 6/31 patients analyzed in the HCTZ/lisinopril group developed severe postpartum hypertension 7 to 10 days after delivery versus 5/36 patients in the extended-release nifedipine group (OR 1.39 95% CI (0.39, 5.01)).

An alternative way to summarize these primary outcomes would be to omit the raw numbers (e.g., 8/30) and just provide ORs and 95% CIs. In this case, however, I think it's wise to include the raw numbers. The CIs are broad (meaning the estimated effects are imprecise) because the sample size in each

---

[9] Rao G. *Rational medical decision making: A case-based approach.* New York: McGraw-Hill, 2006.

group is small. In general, your text summary of primary outcomes will be easier to read if you avoid making it too dense with numerical values.

The next component of the results section is a summary of secondary outcomes and additional and unexpected findings. A large number of outcomes are included on the Clinicaltrials.gov page, but not all of these should be included—for example, there were no maternal deaths. Rare outcomes can be summarized in text form. In such cases, a summary of effect size and precision is often unnecessary. This summary can appear before a table summarizing all key outcomes:

> *Two patients in the HCTZ/lisinopril group developed suffered serious adverse events and were admitted to the ICU compared to zero in the extended-release nifedipine group.*

We know from the Clinicaltrials.gov page that one patient in the HCTZ/lisinopril group developed pulmonary edema, one patient HELLP syndrome, and one patient cardiomyopathy. Since there were three adverse outcomes among two patients, one patient must have suffered more than one adverse outcome, but we can't tell which combination of outcomes she suffered. Best to leave the summary, therefore, as the single sentence above.

The primary and other secondary outcomes can be summarized in a table, appropriately titled "Table 2," along with measures of effect size and precision, as appropriate. Since serious adverse events were so rare (two admissions to the ICU in the HCTZ/lisinopril group), it's fine to leave them out of the table. Table 5.5 shows the outcomes table.

Table 5.5 Sample Outcomes Table

Outcome	HCTZ/ Lisinopril (/n)	Extended-Release Nifedipine (/n)	OR (95% CI)
Stage 2 hypertension/ antihypertensive tx	8/30	12/28	0.48 (0.16, 1.46)
Severe postpartum hypertension	6/31	5/36	1.39 (0.39, 5.01)
Additional antihypertensive tx during admission	6/31	5/36	1.49 (0.40, 5.45)
Median postpartum length of stay in days (interquartile range)	4 (3–5) (n = 31)	3 (3–4) (n = 36)	--
Postpartum readmission	5/31	1/36	6.73 (0.74, 61.1)
Compliant with medications	22/27	26/28	0.88 (0.40, 1.90)

6
The Discussion

The discussion section is either the last or penultimate section of a paper (depending upon if a paper has a separate conclusion section). Its name is quite appropriate: Think of a discussion as the discourse that might take place after consumers of research have read the preceding parts of the paper and meet with the research team. The research consumers would want to go over the main findings and their implications. The format and length of a discussion will vary greatly depending upon the type of research, the journal, and the field. This doesn't mean that you can insert just anything in your discussion; it's not a place for leftover findings or background information you may have omitted in your introduction. Indeed, the discussion has a few clear and distinct purposes:[1]

- To summarize the principal findings of the study (along with unexpected findings)
- To compare the findings to previous similar work
- To summarize strengths and weaknesses of the study
- To provide possible mechanisms or explanation of the findings
- To suggest implications for clinicians and policymakers
- To summarize unanswered questions and suggest areas for future research

What you write in your discussion should fall into one of these six categories. As long as you adhere to this structure, your discussion will be meaningful and impactful. Keep the following principles in mind as well:

1. *Focus on the principal findings or outcomes of your study*. It's tempting to emphasize secondary outcomes if they were significant but the principal outcomes were not. For example, a discussion could begin with "We found the treatment to be effective in patients with a higher baseline

[1] Docherty M, Smith R. The case for structuring the discussion of scientific papers. BMJ 1999 May 8;318(7193):1224–1225. doi:10.1136/bmj.318.7193.1224. PMID: 10231230; PMCID: PMC1115625.

level of pulmonary function." If the study in question enrolled a population with a broad range of pulmonary function, emphasizing the benefits in only a subpopulation would be misleading.

2. *Don't mention new findings in the discussion.* All first mentions of findings belong in the results section. Consider a study of a new therapy for chronic obstructive pulmonary disease (COPD). Including a line such as "Furthermore, in a set of brief interviews, six of the enrollees stated that the new inhaler was easier to use." Yes, it may flow seamlessly into the discussion section, but it's really a finding and thus belongs in the results.

3. *Be respectful in discussing others' prior work.* This seems like common sense, but being sensitive to this principle means a line such as "Unlike the study by Ferguson et al., we enrolled a much more diverse sample of participants" is not the best way to express a difference in study population. It implies that there is something wrong with the way Ferguson et al. carried out their study. Better to state something to the effect of "Our findings may differ from those of Ferguson et al. because they enrolled participants from an area that was racially and ethnically relatively homogeneous." This is a much more respectful way to express a difference since Ferguson et al. may have had no choice but to recruit from an area that was not racially or ethnically diverse.

4. *Avoid exaggerating the implications of your work.* Don't speculate too much about the implications. Stating that "Our groundbreaking therapy is likely to revolutionize treatment for prostate cancer," even if true, may be off-putting to readers. It's much more reasonable to state something like "Our new therapy expands the options available for men with prostate cancer."

Scenario: *Glucagon-like peptide receptor agonists (GLP-1s) have revolutionized treatment of obesity, diabetes, and heart disease. Retatrutide is an emerging weight loss medication that targets three different receptors: GLP-1, glucose-dependent insulinotropic polypeptide (GIP), and glucagon. It has shown promise in promoting weight loss compared to placebo in randomized controlled trials. A natural next step is to compare retatrutide to a widely used GLP-1 receptor agonist. Charles has completed a double-blinded clinical trial among 114 patients comparing retatrutide to semaglutide over a 6-month period, with a primary outcome of percent weight loss. Both medications were titrated up over a 3-month period to a maintenance dose of 12 mg retatrutide and 2.4 mg semaglutide. Table 6.1 shows a complete set of primary and secondary outcomes from the trial.*

Table 6.1 Retatrutide Versus Semaglutide Trial Results

Outcome (means when not specified)	Retatrutide (n = 52)	Semaglutide (n = 56)	P Value for Difference (significant at <0.05)
Change in body weight %, week 12 (SD)	−9.4 (−7.5)	−8.5 (−7.4)	0.08
Change in body weight %, week 26 (SD)	−12.3 (−11.1)	−10.6 (−9.5)	0.06
% patients who lost ≥5% body weight at week 26	76	69	0.09
% patients who lost ≥10% body weight at week 26	42	40	0.10
% patients who lost ≥20% body weight at week 26	8	9	0.27
Mean change in waist circumference at week 26 (cm) (SD)	−8.5 (7.1)	−9.0 (7.2)	0.14
Change in body weight (kg) (SD)	−10.5 (−10.0)	−9.4 (−9.6)	0.12
Change in visceral fat area (%) (SD)	−32.4 (−28.7)	−34.0 (−26.5)	0.18
Change in HbA1C % (SD)	−0.9 (1.1)	−1.0 (1.3)	0.24
Change in systolic blood pressure in mmHg (SD)	−14 (−12)	−6 (−9)	0.03
Change in diastolic blood pressure (mmHg)	−6 (−9)	−2 (−8)	0.03
Number of patients experiencing adverse events	14	12	0.11
Number of patients experiencing adverse events requiring discontinuation	5	1	0.02

What follows is a simple form and some content for the discussion. In reality, there may be lots of unexpected or exciting findings that could be elaborated upon. Charles may also wish to expand the basic findings to provide more quantitative information, though that isn't needed. What I've provided below is just the basics.

Following the basic scheme for a discussion section described earlier, Charles could start with a short paragraph summarizing the principal results of the study. As noted, there is no need to repeat all the results. It's appropriate to state the findings as simple conclusions based on the results:

We found retatrutide and semaglutide to be equally effective in the degree of weight loss at 12 and 26 weeks of treatment, as well as in the proportion of patients who lost 5%, 10%, and 20% of their starting weight at 26 weeks. Retatrutide was associated with a greater reduction in systolic and diastolic blood pressure after 6 months.

Next, Charles could compare his findings to previous work. Retatrutide and semaglutide have never previously been compared head to head, so Charles could discuss if the effects observed were comparable to those from previous studies with placebo or other comparisons.

Our observed effect of retatrutide was not as robust as that observed by Jastreboff et al. in their phase II trial, in which the mean percent weight lost at 8 weeks was 23.9% at a dose of 8 mg retatrutide.[2]

Along with the study above, Charles could also include comparisons with other previous studies. It's important for him to try to explain why the effect of retatrutide in his study may not have been as great as that in the phase II trial.

There were important differences between the sample we recruited and those in the phase II trial. The majority of patients recruited by Jastreboff et al. were men. Seventy-four percent of participants in our study, by contrast, were women. Jastreboff et al. excluded patients with type 2 diabetes. Forty-two percent of enrollees in our study had type 2 diabetes. We are unsure how these factors may have influenced the efficacy of retatrutide.

The observed effect of semaglutide in Charles's study was comparable to that in prior studies, and he should point this out:

In contrast to the diminished effect of retatrutide in our study, the mean effect of semaglutide we observed (10.6% at 26 weeks) was comparable to other semaglutide studies. In a meta-analysis by Qin et al., the mean percent body weight loss with semaglutide versus placebo was 11.8% in trials of 20 to 104 weeks' duration.[3]

---

[2] Jastreboff AM, Kaplan LM, Frías JP, et al. Triple-hormone-receptor agonist retatrutide for obesity: A phase 2 trial. N Engl J Med 2023 Aug 10;389(6):514–526. doi:10.1056/NEJMoa2301972. Epub 2023 Jun 26. PMID: 37366315.

[3] Qin W, Yang J, Deng C, et al. Efficacy and safety of semaglutide 2.4 mg for weight loss in overweight or obese adults without diabetes: An updated systematic review and meta-analysis including the 2-year STEP 5 trial. Diabetes Obes Metab 2024 Mar;26(3):911–923. doi:10.1111/dom.15386. Epub 2023 Nov 28. PMID: 3801;6699.

The next step is to summarize the strengths and weaknesses of the study. Here are some statements Charles could include. Of course, providing more detail about each of these or including additional strengths and weaknesses is perfectly reasonable.

A significant strength of our study is the assessment of the comparative effectiveness of an emerging "triple-G agonist" and an established GLP-1 agonist. Another important strength is the randomized, double-blind design. Our patients were recruited from community settings and included a significant proportion of patients with type 2 diabetes. These are the types of patients likely to benefit most from retatrutide. Recruitment from community, as opposed to hospital or other settings, makes it more likely that our results reflect "real world" conditions in which retatrutide would be prescribed.

Our study has limitations as well. Due to resource limitations, our duration of follow-up was only 6 months. We do not know if retatrutide and semaglutide would be equally effective beyond 6 months. Because of the short duration of our study, doses of retatrutide were titrated from 2 mg to 12 mg weekly, and semaglutide from 0.6 mg to 2.4 mg over a relatively short period of 2 months. A slower rate of titration may be preferable. Our more aggressive approach may explain the relatively high number of adverse events in the retatrutide group. Finally, our patients were recruited from community settings in upstate New York state. 92% of our patients were White. We were not able, therefore, to include a sample that was more representative in terms of race and ethnicity of the United States.

Now it's time for Charles to provide some explanation or mechanism for his findings.

Retatrutide is a triple hormone receptor agonist of the glucose-dependent insulinotropic polypeptide (GIP), glucagon-like peptide 1 (GLP-1), and glucagon receptors (GCG). Semaglutide, by contrast, targets only the GLP-1 receptor. Because of its mechanism of action, one would have expected retatrutide to be more effective in promoting weight loss than semaglutide. Jastreboff et al. speculate that the effect of agonism of the GIP and GLP-1 receptors may be enhanced by activation of GCG receptors. It is possible, however, that one mechanism predominates in promoting weight loss, such that retatrutide is no more effective than a pure GLP-1 agonist. We did, find however, a modest but statistically superior improvement in blood pressure with retatrutide. It's possible, therefore, that retatrutide has superior metabolic and cardiovascular risk reduction effects.

Charles's next step is to suggest implications for clinicians and policymakers. Depending upon the research subject, the type of article, and, most importantly, the actual findings, there may be no such implications. In a basic science article, for example, the implications could include an overall impact on the field such as calling into question certain assumptions that have been made for a long time. There is no formula for writing about implications. Charles could include something like this:

Retatrutide is as effective as semaglutide in promoting weight loss. Our study therefore expands the range of pharmacotherapy available to clinicians who treat obesity. Widespread use of retatrutide in the United States will require recognition of its effectiveness by insurers and policymakers. Given the recent and ongoing surge in demand for weight loss drugs, retatrutide also provides these stakeholders another option to consider.

Finally, Charles needs to summarize unanswered questions that in turn could serve as the basis for future research studies. As a rule, it's important to link this summary to the results of the trial. It's best not to raise unanswered questions that the study was never intended to answer. For example, Charles shouldn't suggest studying the comparative effectiveness of retatrutide exclusively in patients without diabetes. Diabetes was not an exclusion criterion for enrollment, so the effectiveness of retatrutide in patients without diabetes is not a question that emerged directly from the results. By contrast, Charles didn't set out to enroll a sample of patients that was overwhelmingly White; that just happened to be the sample he was able to recruit in upstate New York. Suggesting a more diverse sample for a future study is more reasonable. There are no hard-and-fast rules for this final component of the discussion. Here is a passage Charles could include:

We did not observe the magnitude of effect of retatrutide in our study that was observed in a recent phase II trial. While it's possible that this was because of the characteristics of our sample, it's important to keep in mind that the effectiveness of semaglutide in the same sample was comparable to that shown in prior studies. A useful next step would be to compare retatrutide to another obesity agent in a more racially and ethnically diverse population, and with a sample with a higher proportion of men.

Our study was limited to 6 months' duration. A future study could be much longer in duration. This would allow us to titrate retatrutide and semaglutide (or another agent) more slowly, which may be more effective for weight loss and also minimize side effects.

Our finding of improved blood pressure with retatrutide relative to semaglutide should be replicated in another study. If confirmed, retatrutide may be the preferred agent among patients with obesity and hypertension.

Finally, we are unclear why the triple agonist approach represented by retatrutide was no more effective in promoting weight loss than the GLP-1 agonist. The relative contribution of agonism to each of the three types of receptors is an unresolved question that should be studied further.

The last paragraph clearly stems from the unexpected finding that retatrutide was no more effective than semaglutide in promoting weight loss. However, given that Charles is a clinical trialist, he may not be well positioned to answer this question, which might involve mouse or in vitro studies of some sort. It is simply an interesting call for research to more basic scientists, including those who developed retatrutide.

So there you have it—the basic framework for a discussion. In reality, as noted, a discussion might be considerably longer, especially if there are more unexpected and interesting findings. They key is to include the key elements and to organize your discussion in a logical manner. Table 6.2 describes how the 5Cs are applicable to a discussion section.

Table 6.2 Application of 5Cs to Discussion

Conciseness	Short, sharp sentences will have considerably more impact upon readers than lengthier and more diffuse ones. The discussion is often the longest part of a scientific paper. Overall conciseness, however, is still important. A very long discussion may be difficult for readers to get through. As always, omit needless words and avoid repetition.
Cogency	The active voice is ideal for the discussion, so use it whenever possible—for instance, "We cannot explain" versus "It cannot be explained."
Clarity	Clarity is of great importance in all scientific writing. In a draft of your discussion, make sure each sentence has a clear meaning so that readers don't have to read it twice.
Commonness	It's fine to use jargon in the discussion as long as it appears earlier in some part of the paper. Introducing new terms, acronyms, and so forth in the discussion without explaining them will make the section hard to understand.
Consistency	Follow the general format for a discussion section described in this chapter.

Discussion Exercise

Here is a poorly organized abbreviated discussion section describing an observational study of risk factors for community-acquired pneumonia in children. Your task is to reorganize the discussion (by moving sentences around) using the logical framework discussed in this chapter.

While we were not surprised that smoking in the household was a significant risk factor for community-acquired pneumonia (CAP), it was unexpected that lower parental education was associated with lower risk of CAP. It is possible that parents with lower education are also of lower socioeconomic status and have fewer resources for or less access to care and therefore fewer opportunities to receive a diagnosis of CAP. In other words, many cases of CAP may be missed in lower-income households. Overall, in addition to smoking, we identified history of asthma, incomplete or missing pneumococcal conjugate vaccine, incomplete or missing influenza vaccine, having one or more chronic illnesses such as type 1 diabetes, and obesity as independent risks for CAP. How obesity increases risk for CAP in children is uncertain. It's possible that excess adiposity influences pulmonary function and the ability to clear microorganisms from the lungs. Studying the severity, pulmonary function, and other aspects of CAP among children with obesity would shed light on these issues. The remaining significant risks we identified are expected. Clinicians and policymakers should encourage pneumonia and influenza vaccination among all children, but especially among those with a history of asthma or other chronic illnesses. The risk factors we identified are consistent with those identified in studies by El-Margh et al. and Lucano et al. Lucano et al., in a study of Italian schoolchildren, also identified a history of behavioral problems in school as a risk factor. How undesirable behaviors at school influence the risk for CAP is unknown. Our unexpected finding of a lower level of parental education associated with a lower risk for CAP deserves further study. One approach is to measure school absenteeism for illness among children from lower-parental-education and higher-parental-education households. If absenteeism is comparable or higher among lower-parental-education households, it's possible that these children are getting ill at at least the same rate as children from higher-parental-education households—including with CAP. This would suggest that children from lower-parental-education households interact less with the health system and have fewer opportunities to be diagnosed. Strengths of our study include our large, diverse sample that is reflective of children prone to CAP. Also, we ascertained CAP through multiple means, including electronic health records and insurance claims data. While using multiple methods to confirm a diagnosis is a strength, the use of records rather than radiological findings is a weakness. CAP may be listed as a diagnosis and treated empirically, without radiological confirmation. It's unclear what proportion of children diagnosed with CAP actually have pneumonia, versus another respiratory condition.

Suggested Response

While this lengthy paragraph is easy enough to read, it's not organized in a way that makes the information easy to absorb. Sentences can be simply rearranged according to the framework discussed in this chapter. Though your discussion shouldn't take the form of a table, Table 6.3 provides a scheme for the reorganization.

Not every line from the original passage is included in this reorganization. For example, the original passage describes the association of behavioral problems in school with CAP, but from a different study. The author points out that how behavioral problems influence CAP is uncertain. It would be wise to leave this sentence out because it's not an unexpected finding from the study you're writing a discussion for.

Table 6.3 Reorganized Sentences for Discussion

Summary of principal findings	*Overall, in addition to smoking, we identified a history of asthma, incomplete or missing pneumococcal conjugate vaccine, incomplete or missing influenza vaccine, having one or more chronic illnesses such as type 1 diabetes, and obesity as independent risks for CAP. Children of parents of lower education were less likely to develop CAP.*
Comparison to previous work	*The risk factors we identified are consistent with those identified in studies by El-Margh et al. and Lucano et al. Lucano et al., in a study of Italian schoolchildren, also identified a history of behavioral problems in school as a risk factor.*
Strengths and weaknesses of the study	*Strengths of our study include our large, diverse sample that is reflective of children prone to CAP. Also, we ascertained CAP through multiple means, including electronic health records and insurance claims data. While using multiple methods to confirm a diagnosis is a strength, the use of records rather than radiological findings is a weakness. CAP may be listed as a diagnosis and treated empirically, without radiological confirmation. It's unclear what proportion of children diagnosed with CAP actually have pneumonia, versus another respiratory condition.*
Mechanisms and explanations for findings	*It is possible that parents with lower education are also of lower socioeconomic status and have fewer resources for care or less access to care and therefore fewer opportunities to receive a diagnosis of CAP. How obesity increases risk for CAP in children is uncertain. It's possible that excess adiposity influences pulmonary function and the ability to clear microorganisms from the lungs.*

(continued)

Table 6.3 Continued

Implications for clinicians and policymakers	*Clinicians and policymakers should encourage pneumonia and influenza vaccination among all children, but especially among those with a history of asthma or other chronic illnesses.*
Unanswered questions and areas for future study	*Studying the severity, pulmonary function, and other aspects of CAP among children with obesity would shed light on these issues. (If reorganized should be "shed light on the issue of obesity and its role in CAP.")*
	Our unexpected finding of a lower level of parental education associated with a lower risk for CAP deserves further study. One approach is to measure school absenteeism for illness among children from lower-parental-education and higher-parental-education households. If absenteeism is comparable or higher among lower-parental-education households, it's possible that these children are getting ill at least at the same rate as children from higher-parental-education households— including with CAP. This would suggest that children from lower-parental-education households interact less with the health system and have fewer opportunities to be diagnosed.

7
Writing an Abstract

An abstract is defined as a short and accurate description of a larger body of work. There are different types of biomedical abstracts. The most common use of the term is to describe a published abstract that summarizes a research article. Abstracts are sometimes published in journals or conference proceedings without accompanying research articles, to summarize studies that have been recently completed. An abstract can also refer to a submission to a conference, based on which decisions about opportunities to present the work are made. Abstracts are often required as part of submissions for grants. Yet another form of abstract is a "poster abstract," in which a summary of the work is presented on a poster, together with graphs or charts. All these types of abstracts have much in common, and the principles discussed in this chapter apply to them all. For our purposes, I will refer primarily to abstracts that appear in biomedical journals that summarize the paper they accompany.

An abstract is both unique and important. It's unique because, though it precedes a paper, it is almost always written after all the other parts of the paper have been completed. This is both logical and practical. Key findings and excerpts from the paper can be extracted to help form the abstract. Unfortunately, for many, the abstract is an afterthought—a requirement to which less attention is paid than other parts of the paper. Thinking of an abstract in this way is a big mistake for a number of reasons:

1. The abstract is the part of the paper consumers of research will often read in its entirety before deciding if reading the rest of the paper is worthwhile. A well-written abstract will entice a reader; one that is unclear may discourage the reader.
2. The abstract is used by journal editors and potential reviewers to make initial decisions about a submitted manuscript. As a journal editor, I will read all abstracts submitted with papers to decide if the paper is relevant and the methods are generally sound. If the abstract is poorly written, I suspect the rest of the paper is poorly written as well, and I am inclined not to send it out for review. Reviewers make similar decisions about whether to accept a review task.

3. As accurate summaries of a paper, abstracts are often used to decide if a paper should be included in a systematic review, including quantitative systematic reviews (meta-analyses).
4. In the case of many conference submissions, the abstract is the sole content upon which decisions about acceptance or rejection are made.

Given its overall importance, there are a few important principles and concepts to keep in mind when writing an abstract:

1. Abstracts are sometimes classified as *structured* or *unstructured*. A structured abstract requires specific headings with a couple of sentences under each one. Headings are specified by the journal, conference, or granting body to which you are submitting. Unstructured abstracts do not require such headings and take the form of a single paragraph. Headings for structured abstracts for papers follow a scheme that parallels the paper they describe. The general scheme is background/rationale and aim of the study, methods, results, and conclusions and implications. Different journals prescribe slight variations on this scheme, but the essential required information is largely the same. As a way to stay concise and organized, *I recommend that you write all your abstracts as structured abstracts.* If a journal or other body to which you are submitting prohibits headings, simply remove them and include your structured abstract as a single paragraph without headings. Structured abstracts are simply easier to absorb, and the structure will ensure that you don't miss important information while writing.
2. Both reporting guidelines and organizations such as the International Committee of Medical Journal Editors (ICMJE)[1] provide recommendations on how to write an abstract. Journals, conference, and granting bodies usually provide specific recommendations for abstracts. I have found that these recommendations are sometimes ambiguous. I believe a better strategy for meeting abstract requirements is simply to look at past published abstracts from the same organizations. These are always available for journals and easy to find for other organizations. For example, if I'm considering submitting an abstract to the annual Resuscitation Science Symposium of the American Heart Association, I can easily find submission abstract submissions, such

---

[1] https://www.icmje.org/recommendations/browse/manuscript-preparation/preparing-for-submission.html#b

as this one: https://www.ahajournals.org/doi/10.1161/circ.144.suppl_2.11243.

3. An abstract is a stand-alone description of a body of work. Though the larger body of work will include a great deal of additional detail, an abstract should be complete enough that readers understand the basic purpose, methods, findings, and conclusions found in the larger work. Don't include information in an abstract that can't be found in the larger body of work.

4. Important primary results of research projects are included in an abstract. It's also reasonable to include secondary results if they are especially interesting and space allows.

5. There is no uniform consensus about certain other features of an abstract. In general, it's best to exclude citations. Interested readers can find these in the larger body of work. Include some measure of statistical significance and/or precision with results for key findings. The amount of detail will usually be dictated by the maximum length allowed. Including p-values or confidence intervals for all your primary and secondary results from a research project might lead quickly to an abstract that is too long.

6. Almost all journals and other organizations have strict word limits for abstracts, usually in the range of 200 to 350 words. An abstract should include key information that you believe is important, organized in the way described above. I suggest you first write an abstract that includes everything you believe is important, in a style that is intended to be as comprehensive and descriptive as possible. *Then, while applying the 5Cs, especially conciseness, trim it to the required length.* This will allow you to reflect upon what is most important and what detail is necessary. Aiming to meet the abstract word limits with your first draft, by contrast, makes it more likely you will omit crucial information that needs to be "squeezed in" later. The former approach is easier and will lead to better abstracts.

7. This book is about the craft of scientific writing. It's not about the basics of spelling, grammar, and punctuation. However, pay especially close attention to these areas when writing your abstract. Make your abstract your best possible first impression. An abstract with errors will sour readers on the larger body of work it describes.

<u>Scenario</u>: *Adanna has successfully led a team of researchers in the completion of a qualitative systematic review (i.e., not a meta-analysis) about the effectiveness of structured aerobic exercise programs for the long-term prevention and*

treatment of migraine headaches. She and her team have decided to submit the paper to a general medical journal that requires a structured abstract of 250 words or less. The required abstract sections are background, methods, results, and conclusions. Adanna and her team are also required to add key words that correspond to medical subject headings (MeSH) that will be used to index the paper if it is accepted. (Key words are not included in the word limit.)

What follows is one specific scheme for how the abstract could be written.

The *background* can include the scope of the problem, the rationale for the study, and the specific question being addressed. Some journals will require abstracts with more specific titles than "background" such as "rationale" or "hypothesis." In any case, this section should be no more than two or three sentences. Here's what Adanna came up with:

Though pharmacological treatment is often effective in the prevention and treatment of migraine headache, many migraine sufferers experience medication side effects, prefer non-pharmacological approaches for other reasons, or have residual symptoms despite treatment with medication. Structured aerobic exercise is a non-pharmacological treatment that has shown promise in individual studies, but reported results of effectiveness vary considerably or are conflicting. Our goal was to identify the overall effectiveness of structured aerobic exercise for the prevention and treatment of migraine headache. (80 words)

Adanna's background is quite clear, but using up 80 words, or roughly one-third of her allocated limit, means it will likely require trimming. As noted above, she should worry about that later. Note the use of the past tense and the active voice, which are preferred in most situations.

Here is the methods section of her abstract:

We searched the following electronic databases for randomized controlled trials published between 2018 and 2025 of structured aerobic exercise programs with or without medication treatment compared to usual care or no treatment among chronic migraine sufferers: the Cochrane Central Register of Controlled Trials (CENTRAL), MEDLINE, Embase, and PsycINFO. We also searched Google Scholar as well as the reference lists of all retrieved citations for additional papers. Abstracts of all papers were reviewed by a minimum of two authors who decided to include a paper. Disagreements were settled by a third author. Papers that described unstructured exercise programs and other forms of exercise (e.g., yoga) were excluded. We limited our search to papers published in English and those in which the population included adults. Methodological quality of included papers was assessed using the Cochrane risk-of-bias tool. (135 words)

Again, Adanna's description of methods is reasonably well-written, but at 135 words, it is simply too long and will require trimming.

Here is her draft results section:

Our initial search yielded 124 articles. We excluded 115 of these for various reasons including interventions that were unstructured or completely patient self-directed, inclusion of participants with unspecified headache types, comparison to other lifestyle programs (e.g., relaxation therapy), and high risk of bias. Among the nine studies we included, seven reported a significant and meaningful benefit of structured aerobic exercise with or without medication upon migraine frequency and severity of symptoms. Four studies reported a positive impact upon quality of life. No studies reported negative or adverse effects of structured aerobic exercise. (92 words)

Adanna's abstract is for a qualitative systematic review. It's not unusual to omit quantitative information (e.g., improvement in headache scores) from such abstracts. She could also have given a range of improvement, but that's not always possible since different studies may use different outcome measures. Results from the individual studies were not pooled (i.e., "meta-analyzed"), likely due to heterogeneity in the duration and other characteristics of the exercise programs, differences in populations, and differences in outcomes.

Finally, Adanna needs a *conclusion*. One sentence is ideal, though two is acceptable:

The majority of studies included in this systematic review report a beneficial effect of structured aerobic exercise for the prevention and treatment of migraine, either alone or in combination with medications. When available, structured aerobic exercise should be offered to migraine sufferers. (42 words)

Adanna's total abstract is 349 words, well above the 250-word limit. If ever there was a need for conciseness in scientific writing, it is in writing an abstract. She considered two strategies to shorten the abstract: omitting needless words and omitting unnecessary detail that can be found in the body of the manuscript. Since her abstract is nearly 50% too long, it's reasonable to try and cut about a third of each section.

Here is what she did with the background section:

Original: *Though pharmacological treatment is often effective in the prevention and treatment of migraine headache, many migraine sufferers experience medication side effects, prefer non-pharmacological approaches for other reasons, or have residual symptoms despite treatment with medication. Structured aerobic exercise is a non-pharmacological treatment that has shown promise in individual studies, but reported results of effectiveness vary considerably or are conflicting. Our goal was to identify the overall effectiveness of structured aerobic exercise for the prevention and treatment of migraine headache.* (80 words)

Revised: *Medications are effective for treatment of migraine but can be inadequately effective and associated with side effects. Many sufferers prefer non-pharmacological approaches. Structured aerobic exercise has shown promising but highly variable results. Our goal was to estimate the effectiveness of structured aerobic exercise for the prevention and treatment of migraine.* (50 words)

There is no precise formula for shortening this and the other sections, apart from asking if each word and detail is necessary. Simply having a target number of words is helpful in identifying what can be eliminated.

Adanna continues in the same way with the methods section:

Original: *We searched the following electronic databases for randomized controlled trials published between 2018 and 2025 of structured aerobic exercise programs with or without medication treatment compared to usual care or no treatment among chronic migraine sufferers: the Cochrane Central Register of Controlled Trials (CENTRAL), MEDLINE, Embase, and PsycINFO. We also searched Google Scholar as well as the reference lists of all retrieved citations for additional papers. Abstracts of all papers were reviewed by a minimum of two authors who decided to include a paper. Disagreements were settled by a third author. Papers that described unstructured exercise programs and other forms of exercise (e.g., yoga) were excluded. We limited our search to papers published in English and those in which the population included adults. Methodological quality of included papers was assessed using the Cochrane risk-of-bias tool.* (135 words)

Revised: *We searched for papers published in English in CENTRAL, MEDLINE, Embase, PsycINFO, and Google scholar from 2018 to 2025 for randomized trials among adults of structured aerobic exercise programs with or without medications compared to usual care or no treatment. We also searched reference lists of retrieved papers. Two authors reviewed abstracts to decide about inclusion, with a third settling disagreements. Quality was assessed with the Cochrane risk-of-bias tool.* (69 words)

Her revised methods section is only about half the length of the original. Notice that in addition to eliminated needless words, Adanna has left out exclusion criteria; readers can easily find this detail in the body of the paper. Also, the acronym for CENTRAL is not spelled out, which is consistent with the other listed database acronyms.

As she has been quite successful with the first two sections, there is less trimming required for the results and conclusion. Nevertheless, here are her original and revised results sections:

Original: *Our initial search yielded 124 articles. We excluded 115 of these for various reasons including interventions that were unstructured or completely patient self-directed, inclusion of participants with unspecified headache types, comparison to other lifestyle programs (e.g., relaxation therapy), and high risk of bias. Among the nine studies we included, seven reported a significant and meaningful benefit of structured aerobic exercise with or without medication upon migraine frequency and severity of symptoms. Four studies reported a positive impact upon quality of life. No studies reported negative or adverse effects of structured aerobic exercise.* (92 words)

Revised: *We excluded 115 of 124 articles from our initial search because they described unstructured or self-directed programs, included patients with unspecified headache types, compared interventions to other lifestyle programs (e.g., relaxation therapy) or had high risk of bias. Seven of nine studies reported a significant benefit of structured aerobic exercise with or without medication upon migraine frequency and severity. Four reported a positive impact upon quality of life and none reported adverse effects.* (73 words)

Adanna's results section is trimmed modestly. Notice the elimination of some superfluous words—"negative" and "adverse" mean essentially the same thing in this context, for example.

Finally, here are her original and revised conclusions:

Original: *The majority of studies included in this systematic review report a beneficial effect of structured aerobic exercise for the prevention and*

treatment of migraine, either alone or in combination with medications. When available, structured aerobic exercise should be offered to migraine sufferers.
(42 words)

<u>Revised</u>: *Either alone or in combination with medications, structured aerobic exercise has been shown in the majority of studies to be beneficial for the prevention and treatment of migraine, and, when available, should be offered.*
(34 words)

There was no need for Adanna to revise her conclusion at all to meet the 250-word requirement. It is, nevertheless, a good practice to keep abstracts short while retaining essential information, which is what her revision does. The total abstract is now only 226 words. She could add back information (such as exclusion criteria) or add in additional detail. An abstract that is well under the word limit is also perfectly fine.

Adanna needs a few key words that will help index her paper in electronic databases correctly. She chooses "migraine," "aerobic exercise," and "systematic review." As noted, for the journal to which she is submitting, these are not included in the abstract word limit.

Table 7.1 describes the application of the 5Cs to writing an abstract.

Table 7.1 Application of the 5Cs to Abstracts

Conciseness	Conciseness is obviously essential for writing an abstract. Follow the example of Adanna's abstract above. As you aim to meet the word limit, always ask if each word and detail is necessary.
Cogency	Use the active voice in your abstract unless the journal or other organization you are submitting to specifies otherwise.
Clarity	Given how important an abstract is in decisions to review, publish, or accept for a conference or funding opportunity, make sure each sentence is absolutely clear. Check for ambiguity by reading each sentence several times and considering how it may be interpreted other than intended. Always get someone not involved in the work to read your abstract to make sure they understand it the same way you do.
Commonness	Avoiding jargon is generally important, but it's actually OK *not* to spell out some common acronyms to save space. A couple of examples: COPD (chronic obstructive pulmonary disease) and ESRD (end-stage renal disease).
Consistency	Like conciseness, consistency is essential for an abstract. Follow the headings and other format requirements specified in the journal or other entity to which you are submitting. Even when unstructured abstracts are acceptable, structure your abstract based on the conventions in this chapter and remove headings.

Abstract Exercise

Your task is to shorten this 339-word abstract to 100 words or less. The title of this article is "Randomized Trial of Mobile Phone Application for Smoking Cessation."

Background: *Cigarette smoking remains a significant public health problem. More than 15% of American adults smoke. Smoking is associated not only with chronic obstructive pulmonary disease but also heart disease. It is also associated with lung cancer and a number of other malignancies. Counseling and medications can be effective in helping smokers quit but are sometimes inaccessible due to cost or availability. By contrast, the vast majority of adults have access to a smartphone, and smartphone-based apps have been shown to be effective in the self-management of chronic illnesses. Smartphone-based applications are also often more convenient and less expensive to deliver than other types of smoking-cessation interventions. Our principal aim was to evaluate the effectiveness of a smartphone-based application for smoking cessation in a randomized controlled trial compared to an in-person counseling program (control intervention).*

Methods: *Eligible participants were recruited from primary care practices and community locations in various ways, including direct referral by physicians, health fairs, and other community events. Eligibility requirements included the following: age ≥ 18 years, not currently engaged in a quit attempt, smoking a minimum of 10 cigarettes daily most days of the week, access to and able to use a smartphone application. The smartphone application was based on acceptance and commitment therapy (ACT). Participants were asked to download it, set a quit date, and received education about its use during a short in-person session. Control group participants received three in-person sessions, each lasting 30 minutes, and delivered by a trained smoking cessation counselor in an easily accessible community location over the course of 1 month. The primary outcome was 3-month self-reported abstinence.*

Results: *We recruited 116 participants. Sixty were assigned to the smartphone app arm, and 56 to the control arm. Among the 60 assigned to the smartphone app, 28 reported abstinence at 3 months, compared to 16 in the control arm who reported abstinence at 3 months (odds ratio, 1.45, 95% CI 1.21, 1.77).*

Conclusion: *A smartphone-based application for smoking cessation is superior to a three-session in-person counseling program in promoting abstinence after 3 months.*

Suggested Response

There are many opportunities to trim this abstract. The background is too lengthy. The hazards of cigarette smoking are well known, as is the usefulness of counseling and medications and the advantages of smartphone applications, especially to someone with an interest in the paper. These statements can be omitted. There are many sentences that repeat elements or are embellished in different ways. "Odds ratio" can be simply written as in its well-known form "OR." There is no single correct way to trim the abstract, but here is one possibility that cuts the word count to 96 words, headings included:

Background: *Mobile applications are useful in self-management of chronic disease. Our aim was to compare a smartphone-based app to an in-person counseling program (control) for smoking cessation.*

Methods: *Adult smokers were randomized to a smartphone app based on acceptance and commitment therapy (ACT) or to three 30-minute counseling sessions. The primary outcome was self-reported abstinence at 3 months.*

Results: *28 of 60 patients in the smartphone group and 16/56 in the control group were abstinent (OR 1.45, 95% CI, 1.21, 1.77).*

Conclusion: *A smartphone-based app is more effective than a three-session counseling program for smoking cessation.*

8
Grant Writing

Good Ideas Expressed Poorly

I have been a reviewer on a study section for the Agency for Healthcare Research and Quality (AHRQ) for several years and have reviewed, scored, and led discussions of hundreds of grant proposals. AHRQ funds research projects in broad areas of health services research including patient safety, implementation of recommendations from research studies, and quality improvement. The procedures and policies through which grants are awarded are identical in many respects to those of the National Institutes of Health (NIH). There is one important thing all research granting bodies have in common, be they in the United States, Canada, Europe, or elsewhere—*It's awfully difficult to obtain a grant.* The number of grant applications these organizations receive is far greater than the funds they have available. Grant funding is therefore a highly competitive, if not brutal, process, with which I'm personally very familiar. It took me years of successive attempts through multiple applications and ideas to obtain my first federal research grant. Succeeding is a matter of selling an idea to a group of reviewers whose mission is to scrutinize your proposal as carefully as possible. As a reviewer, I've learned over the years that nothing can rescue a bad idea, no matter how well a proposal is written. The likelihood of funding for a good idea, however, is seriously compromised if the proposal is poorly written. Countless times have I read a proposal whose underlying concept is sound, but I just can't figure out precisely what the applicant is trying to say, or the application is so disorganized that it makes me question the applicant's commitment to putting his or her best idea forward.

The focus of this book and this chapter is on writing. I obviously can't help you if your idea isn't sound. Always aim to be in the right-bottom box of the matrix in Table 8.1.

Just how difficult is to get funded? Let's first consider the NIH as an example, as the institutes are collectively by far the largest biomedical granting organization in the world. The NIH defines "success rate" as the percent of

Table 8.1 Likelihood of Funding for a Grant Proposal

	Poor Idea	Excellent Idea
Poor quality of writing	Low success rate	Low success rate
High quality of writing	Low success rate	High success rate

peer-reviewed applications that receive funding.[1] Success rates are calculated for each fiscal year. So if you submit a proposal, receive a review, and then re-submit a revised version of the proposal in the same fiscal year, it is counted only once in the success rate. In 2023, the NIH received 51,883 research grant applications, of which 11,052 (21.3%) received funding.[2]

Keep in mind that conceptualizing, writing, and assembling an NIH grant of any kind is a substantial endeavor that requires excellent organizational and leadership skills. The process of grant writing for me begins months in advance of the submission deadline, many meetings with team members, countless revisions, and a huge number of hours that sometimes compromises my other professional activities such as patient care, ongoing research, or teaching. Successful or not, most applicants make the same sort of effort. The fact that nearly 80% fail despite this huge effort is daunting. Success rates from other bodies and in other countries are comparable. The Canadian Institutes Health Research (CIHR) funded just 17.2% of applications in 2023. The rate in the United Kingdom is comparable.[3]

Of course, 80% of grant applications aren't rejected on the basis of poor writing alone. There is lots of advice about grant writing and many lists of common mistakes in writing grants, including one from the National Institute of Mental Health (NIMH).[4] Most of these shortcomings can be classified under (1) a lack of potential impact of the proposed research or (2) missing information or lack of detail in one or more areas. There are also the problems of overly ambitious aims, investigators without the requisite experience or expertise, and failure to follow basic instructions. You won't usually find a lack of clarity in writing or the other 5Cs listed or referred to in these widely available lists of grant mistakes.

---

[1] https://report.nih.gov/sites/report/files/2023-12/NIH%20Success%20Rates%20Definition.pdf. Accessed May 17, 2024.

[2] https://nexus.od.nih.gov/all/2024/02/21/fy-2023-by-the-numbers-extramural-grant-investments-in-research/. Accessed May 17, 2024.

[3] Sathian B, van Teijlingen E, Banerjee I, Kabir R. Guidance to applying for health research grants in the UK. Nepal J Epidemiol 2022 Dec 31;12(4):1231–1234. doi:10.3126/nje.v12i4.50998. PMID: 36741773; PMCID: PMC98886560.

[4] https://www.nimh.nih.gov/funding/grant-writing-and-application-process/common-mistakes-in-writing-applications. Accessed May 17, 2024.

Let's start with the assumption that your idea is sound and potentially impactful; that you have provided all the information reviewers might need; that you have the required experience and expertise to complete the proposed work, which is reasonable in scope; and that you followed all submission requirements. What you are left with is the task of selling your sound idea to a group of reviewers. This is when the writing becomes really important. I'll describe my own experience as a reviewer in this regard.

In advance of a study section, I'm typically asked to review and score between five and seven grants. These are sent to me about 4 weeks in advance of the study section meeting. I spend an average of 4 to 5 hours on each one. Some reviewers spend less time; others, considerably more. Reviewing grants isn't a full-time activity for anyone—I have to squeeze these roughly 30 hours into my other professional and personal activities. For me, these include a great deal of writing (sometimes grants), editing, and reviewing other materials, not to mention other scholarly reading and writing clinical notes. Basically, like most physicians in academic settings, I read and write a great deal every day. Additional time and energy to scrutinize a grant proposal is always scarce.

In reviewing a proposal, a poorly conceived idea or one that includes the other mistakes I've described takes some time to uncover. In fact, I'm often initially excited by the "specific aims" page and am enthusiastic about reading the rest of the proposal. Only after reflecting, doing a bit of my own research, or more carefully looking for potentially missing information will I decide that a grant shouldn't be scored highly. If a grant is well written, I will arrive at this point of careful reflection after a few hours. A poorly written proposal, by contrast, won't even make it that far—not with me, and not with most reviewers.

If the first sentence I read is ambiguous or makes no sense, my mindset changes immediately from one of curiosity and enthusiasm to simply being annoyed. I anticipate that reading the rest of the grant will be a chore. As a writer and editor, I become more vigilant to additional problems with the writing, which means, by necessity, that I pay less attention to the science and other aspects of the proposal. I can tell you from experience that poor writing has a similar impact on my fellow reviewers—it puts us all in a foul mood. As a grant writer you want to make sure your proposal makes it to the point that the science is being considered thoroughly and fairly. The writing needs to be clear, bold, and organized to get to that point.

To hammer this point home, consider a study by Peter van den Besselian and Charlin Mom entitled "The Effect of Writing Style on Success in Grant Applications."[5] Theirs is a complex study that makes heavy use of the lexicon of

---

[5] Van den Besselaar P, Mom C. The effect of writing style on success in grant applications. J Informetrics 2022;16(1):101257.

linguistics. Nevertheless, based on analysis of 2,532 European grant proposals, they were able to draw some meaningful conclusions that you should consider in writing proposals.

First, they conclude simply that "writing style matters." In Europe, for the grant schemes they evaluated, applicants who make it through a first round of review are often invited to present to a panel to further explain their proposed work and answer questions. Van den Besselian and Mom describe these presentations as "stage performance," an important activity in addition to making sure the science in a proposal is sound. In most settings, the equivalent of a stage performance for a grant proposal is the writing style—how neatly and persuasively it is put together, as opposed to the soundness of the science. Stage performance, whether written or as a presentation, matters, and specific aspects of writing are more likely to be associated with success in obtaining funding. Second, proposals that demonstrate higher English proficiency, more causal language (use of strong claims and certainty in language, aligned with "cogency"), and short sentences are scored higher. Third, proposals that follow a more narrative rather than an analytic style are scored higher. Analytic writing dominates scientific prose and includes many facts and explanations. A narrative style is more like a story. Constructing a grant proposal as a persuasive story is more compelling for reviewers. I'll describe a couple of examples later in this chapter.

Overall, in contrast to making sure your ideas are scientifically sound and organized according to requirements, about which there is a great deal of advice available, there is very little advice about writing style such as in Van den Besselaar's and Mom's paper. Robert Porter offers additional meaningful advice in his paper entitled "Why Academics Have a Hard Time Writing Good Grant Proposals," which won best paper at a research administration conference where it was presented.[6] Porter contrasts what he calls "academic writing," or the writing found in scholarly papers, to the writing in successful grant proposals. He states, "Success in grant writing is a matter of style and format as much as content." Porter makes several important points. Readers of a paper are more likely to have a strong interest and expertise in its topic; grant reviewers, by contrast, though they may have a general interest in the overall field of a set of grant proposals, are unlikely to have the same degree of expertise. This of course means that a grant proposal has to be easier to understand, must use simpler language, and must also explain terms or concepts with which reviewers are likely to be unfamiliar. A paper uses "expository rhetoric" or "explaining to the reader" as opposed to "persuasive rhetoric" or

---

[6] Porter R. Why academics have a hard time writing good grant proposals. J Res Admin 2007;38:37–43.

"selling the reader." Clarity and conciseness are crucial. Of the writing in grant proposals, Porter states, "Sentences are shorter, with key phrases underlined or bolded to make them stand out. Lists are printed bullet style. Graphs, table and drawings abound. . . . The writing is more energetic, direct and concise."

Porter's best advice, in my opinion, is to emulate the style of writing found in *Scientific American*, in which world-class scientists explain complicated subjects to a highly educated audience that is nevertheless usually unfamiliar with the subjects. Here is an excerpt from a *Scientific American* article on the impact of high summer temperatures on the immune system:[7]

> *A team of scientists recently untangled how short-term heat exposure affects the body's defense network in a study presented at a conference in Chicago that was held by the American Heart Association in March. The researchers took one-time blood samples from 624 individuals in Louisville, Ky., as temperatures fluctuated in the summers of 2018 and 2019, and they analyzed various immune molecules that served as biomarkers for inflammation and an immune response. The average temperature when the blood draws occurred was a balmy 75 degrees Fahrenheit (24 degrees Celsius), with most temperatures falling between 69 and 80 degrees F (21 and 27 degrees C), yet the researchers found a sweep of inflammatory changes among study participants on the days that were warmer than average, suggesting that even mild heat was causing the immune system to go into fight mode and expend valuable resources. These findings have researchers considering long-term consequences of rapidly rising global temperatures on immune function.*

Fairly easy to understand, isn't it? If you are new to proposal writing, I urge you to read a few articles in *Scientific American* to learn how to make your writing as easy to understand for reviewers.

Another critical step in writing a proposal is to review prior successful grant applications for the same or similar program or institution. This, of course, will not only give you a good idea about how a proposal should be written but will also provide helpful information about format, organization, and sponsor priorities. Assuming you have an excellent and sound idea, follow all format requirements, and have made sure your idea is aligned with the sponsor's priorities, before writing a word, carefully review at least one prior successful application. The National Cancer Institute (NCI), for examples, offers sample

---

[7] https://www.scientificamerican.com/article/the-immune-system-may-struggle-to-handle-hotter-summer-temperatures/. Accessed May 20, 2024.

applications here: https://cancercontrol.cancer.gov/is/funding/sample-grant-applications.

Even if you can't easily find a prior successful application online, there is nothing wrong with asking the sponsor or funding agency for a sample application or asking an investigator or team that has been successful to share their grant. You will learn a great deal about successful grant writing simply by emulating the style of prior successful proposals. Let's consider one example of a successful NCI application entitled "Predicting and Addressing Colonoscopy Non-adherence in Community Settings," available here: https://healthcaredelivery.cancer.gov/funding/samples.html. Dr. Coronado's proposal is both scientifically sound and superbly written. One of the principles discussed above is to write more narratively and less analytically. This advice is hard to apply without a concrete example. Take a look at the headings in the Significance section of the proposal on page 7. Notice that the headings outline a compelling story: "Many patients . . . forgo colonoscopies," "Colonoscopy follow-up rates vary," "Colonoscopy follow-up rates in community health centers are suboptimal," "Patient navigation is a promising approach," and "Despite promise, more information is needed to best target patient navigation resources." The order is logical, and a story clearly emerges that explains the importance of the proposed research. This is the type of writing you should aim for.

In addition to the 5Cs, which are applicable to all scientific writing, I recommend the following:

1. Your grant should read like a well-written story, starting with your aims and then progressing through background/significance and approach.
2. Unlike in a scientific paper, repetition is perfectly acceptable. For example, you might state that "Asthma is a serious . . ." in the aims section; then mention it again, quoting statistics, in the background section; and then subtly again in the approach section: "Given how serious and common asthma is . . ."
3. Cogency is necessary overall. Use the active voice as much as possible. Use bold language. Be persuasive.
4. After your idea is well developed, you have sufficient preliminary data, you have reviewed grant requirements, you have planned your grant writing well in advance of the submission date, you have confirmed interest from the sponsor with a program or grants officer, etc., review at least three successful proposals. Also spend a few hours reviewing articles in *Scientific American*, preferably on the same or similar subject. The writing style will have a conscious or even unconscious impact on how you write your proposal.

Exercise

This exercise is designed to give you experience with the style and tone of grant proposal writing.

1. Follow the link below, which will take you to a 2019 *British Medical Journal* article comparing pulmonary rehabilitation provided through telemedicine with normal or usual care pulmonary rehabilitation in a randomized trial. The study was carried out in Denmark. Read the abstract, introduction, and methods section to familiarize yourself with the study and its most important results: https://thorax.bmj.com/content/75/5/413.long.
2. Imagine that it's 2014. You believe telemedicine pulmonary rehabilitation is a promising alternative to regular rehabilitation because it can be delivered less expensively and is more convenient for patients. You are seeking funding for the study above. Your goal is to write a very short capsule summary of your proposal, no longer than 100 words. It should read like a sales pitch for your study and should include a clear description of the problem and what is unknown. It should end with your idea to fill the gap in knowledge. You may wish to add a couple of citations describing the scope of the problem and the promise of telemedicine rehabilitation (you can search for these at PubMed.com). Citations don't count toward the word limit. Apply the four recommendations in the list I described earlier.
3. Read your 100-word pitch to a colleague and ask them if they understand the importance of the study and what you wish to accomplish.

Suggested Response

This isn't an easy exercise, due partly to the limited prescribed length of the piece and also the need to adopt a more narrative and persuasive style than you would use in a manuscript submitted to a journal. There are many ways to write the piece, including this one:

Nearly one in five patients with COPD have severe or very severe disease.[8]
Along with a number of other treatments such as medications, pulmonary

---

[8] Bednarek M, Maciejewski J, Wozniak M, et al. Prevalence, severity and underdiagnosis of COPD in the primary care setting. Thorax 2008 May;63(5):402–407. doi:10.1136/thx.2007.085456. Epub 2008 Jan. 30. PMID: 18234906.

rehabilitation has been shown to offer benefit to such patients.[9] *Unfortunately, formal rehabilitation programs are underused due to their inconvenience, especially for patients with limited mobility. They are also very expensive or unavailable in many places. Rehabilitation provided by telemedicine is a promising alternative that can overcome these barriers.*[10] *However, we don't know if it is as effective as traditional rehabilitation. Our goal is to compare the two approaches in a randomized trial.*

This paragraph, which is 97 words long, provides a short summary of the scope of the problem, the shortcomings of regular pulmonary rehabilitation, the gap in knowledge, and what the proposal is trying to accomplish. While persuasiveness is difficult to convey in such a short paragraph, the order of sentences is logical and the paragraph presents a compelling story.

---

[9] Rochester CL, Alison JA, Carlin B, et al. Pulmonary rehabilitation for adults with chronic respiratory disease: An official American Thoracic Society Clinical Practice Guideline. Am J Respir Crit Care Med 2023 Aug 15;208(4):e7–e26. doi:10.1164/rccm.202306-1066ST. PMID: 37581410; PMCID: PMC10449064.
[10] Bryant MS, Bandi VD, Nguyen CK, et al. Telehealth pulmonary rehabilitation for patients with severe chronic obstructive pulmonary disease. Fed Pract 2019 Sep;36(9):430–435. PMID: 31571812; PMCID: PMC6752812.

9

Grant Writing

Specific Aims

The specific aims section is an important component of applications for grants to the National Institutes of Health (NIH), the Agency for Healthcare Research and Quality, and many other governmental and non-governmental funding agencies in the United States. The specific aims section, while sometimes called something else, is also a necessary component of research grant submissions in other countries as well, such as the United Kingdom.[1] Moreover, a well-written specific aims page is considered by many to be the most important part of a research grant application. Santen et al. have even described it as the "jewel in the crown" of an investigator-initiated proposal.[2] There is a clear reason for this: Obtaining funding from bodies such as the NIH is a highly competitive process in which experienced researchers are tasked with reviewing grant submissions and discussing their merits and shortcomings in a group meeting. Each reviewer, as I discussed earlier based on my own experience, receives roughly five to seven proposals shortly before a meeting. At the study section meeting, it's my job (along with two additional reviewers of each of the same proposals) to describe the strengths and weaknesses of each proposal. The reviews and the study section assessment greatly influence the likelihood of funding.

Grant proposals can be lengthy and dense. Many are highly technical in their content and can be difficult to understand for reviewers whose own field is not well aligned. This is why the specific aims page is so important. The page summarizes the problem to be tackled, what is already known, what the researcher is proposing, the overall objective of the research, and the specific objectives or aims to be accomplished. It takes just a few minutes to read a specific aims page, and, if it is well written, the reviewer will get a very nice idea of

---

[1] NHR Work and Health Research Collaboration Awards Stage 1 Guidance for Applicants. https://www.nihr.ac.uk/documents/nihr-work-and-health-research-collaboration-awards-stage-1-guidance-for-applicants/35019. Accessed December 27, 2023.

[2] Santen RJ, Barrett EJ, Siragy HM, et al. The jewel in the crown: Specific aims section of investigator-initiated grant proposals. J Endocr Soc 2017;1(9):1194–1202.

the importance and practicalities of the proposed research. Given the work-load each reviewer faces, a well-written specific aims page is the researcher's best opportunity to engage and excite a reviewer about the proposed research. Monte and Libby from the University of Colorado write, "Although a grant cannot be won with the Specific Aims page, a proposal can be lost on there by confusing or alienating reviewers."[3]

Whether or not you plan to submit a research grant proposal or have experience in writing key components including specific aims, writing an effective specific aims page is an excellent writing exercise in being clear, concise, and persuasive.

The Fundamentals

The specific aims section may take slightly different forms, with different requirements depending upon the funding agency and the country in which it is based. There are, however, some common general recommendations.

First, your specific aims page should be just that—a single page. There are lots of websites available as well as journal articles describing what to include in the specific aims page. Some provide highly specific recommendations for the number of sentences and the content of each. Most resources recommend a page consisting of four paragraphs: an introduction; a body paragraph; the actual aims, usually accompanied by hypotheses; and, finally, an impact paragraph summarizing the potential impact on the field of the proposed research.

The introductory paragraph should clearly define the problem to be addressed, why the problem is significant, what is already known about the area of research, and what gap or gaps in knowledge remain, and then closes by describing the critical need to fill the gap or gaps in research. The first sentence is crucial—reviewers need to be persuaded that the problem to be addressed is important.

The second or "body" paragraph is typically more detailed and includes the solution to the critical need the research team is proposing, and the ra-tionale for the solution. It also may include why the research team is qualified to tackle the problem, as well as a brief summary of any preliminary data that would support the proposal. The body paragraph also includes the long-term goal or objective of the research. The paragraph should conclude with a cen-tral, overarching hypothesis testable by the aims.

---

[3] Monte AA, Libby AM. Introduction to the specific aims page of a grant proposal. Acad Emerg Med 2018;25(9):1042–1047.

The third paragraph includes the actual specific aims, usually two or three in number. Each aim tests part of the central hypothesis and describes what will be accomplished. Aims for investigator-initiated research proposals are often each accompanied by an explicitly stated hypothesis to be tested.

The final paragraph is the payoff paragraph and develops advocacy for your proposal among reviewers. It should include a description of the overall significance, innovativeness, and impact of the proposed research, including how it will advance the field by expanding knowledge or changing practice.

These four paragraphs constitute the basic structure of the specific aims page. There are many variations. For example, sometimes "sub-aims" are included under each specific aim. Sometimes explicit hypotheses are not included for each aim. Let's ignore these variations for now and focus upon the simplest and most common structure. Also, let's not worry about whether the project described in the following scenario is truly innovative or useful, nor whether the project is worthy of research funding. This book is about writing well, not about perfectly sound research ideas. So, let's get started.

Scenario: *Madison ("Maddie") is a pediatrician working in a primary care center in a large academic center. Her patients come mostly from poor, minority families in an economically challenged area of a large city. Over the years she has developed a strong interest in improving care for children and adolescents with asthma. She has seen many of her patients wind up in the emergency room with asthma exacerbations, often with severe symptoms. Sadly, one of her adolescent patients died of an asthma attack in 2022.*

Maddie would like to improve ongoing care for children and adolescents with asthma to prevent severe exacerbations and treatment in the hospital. Peak flow (PF) is measured by inspiring fully and then blowing out as hard and as fast as possible into the mouthpiece of a device known as a PF meter. Decreases in PF are known to occur prior to worsening symptoms. Regular PF monitoring, therefore, can prevent exacerbations and hospitalizations.

In her routine care, in addition to emphasizing the importance of influenza vaccination and avoidance of cigarette smoke, Maddie encourages all her patients who are old enough to regularly monitor their PF and to self-manage their asthma in a dynamic fashion based on PF values.

While this is all fine in theory, Maddie has struggled to encourage her patients and their parents to monitor PF regularly at home, even though PF meters are inexpensive and widely available. Patients often forget to do so, and, even when they do, real-time advice isn't available.

Together with two engineering colleagues, Maddie has developed a new type of PF meter (GuideFlow) that connects to a smart phone via Bluetooth and includes an easy-to-use smartphone app. GuideFlow informs patients if an appropriate effort was made with the forced expiration and the recorded value is therefore usable and if PF has decreased compared to the patient's usual number. It also makes recommendations about what to do in such cases based on a management plan given to each patient by his or her physician (e.g., double the dose of steroid inhaler for the next 2 days). GuideFlow also reminds users to measure PF twice daily (in the morning and in the afternoon).

GuideFlow was developed through pilot technology funding. Maddie also tested it for a week among 20 of her own patients who were surveyed afterwards and reported that the device and app were easy to use. She is ready to apply for an NIH grant for a study to implement GuideFlow in a randomized trial, comparing it to a standard PF meter accompanied by written instructions.

To begin, Maddie needs a cogent first sentence to get reviewers' attention and immediately make clear the importance of the problem she wishes to address. Here are a few ways she might begin her specific aims page; let's consider each in sequence.

The prevalence of asthma among children and adolescents is steadily increasing.

Not a bad way to begin. Certainly, many review articles about asthma might start the same way, but this is hardly eye-catching.

What about this one?

Despite a well-established recommendation for regular peak-flow monitoring among patients with asthma, rates of such self-monitoring among children and adolescents are suboptimal.

While this seems like a clear beginning sentence, it's not very cogent. You have the advantage of knowing what Maddie wants to study and some idea of how she plans to go about it, but imagine that you didn't have that insight and are a reviewer (perhaps unfamiliar with asthma care). If you read that first sentence, would you struggle to understand it? Would it grab your attention?

Now keeping in mind the 5Cs, especially cogency, consider this one:

Too many poor children are hospitalized or die from asthma.

You don't need to know anything about peak flow or asthma guidelines to understand that one. It's a bold statement—a conclusion that grabs enough of your attention to encourage you to read on. To support it, Maddie could include statistics from a research paper. Her next task is to describe in one or two sentences what is known about the problem, including the benefits of regular PF monitoring. A nice way for her to begin overall could be:

> Too many poor children are hospitalized or die from asthma. In 2024, more than 700,000 children were admitted to emergency rooms or inpatient facilities with asthma exacerbations. There were more than 3,000 asthma-related deaths among children, a number that has been steadily increasing. Asthma self-management has been shown to reduce asthma exacerbations and therefore asthma-related morbidity and mortality. Regular peak-flow (PF) monitoring is an important, widely recommended component of asthma self-monitoring. Unfortunately, most children, including those at higher risk for asthma morbidity and mortality such as minority children and children from poor families, do not monitor PF regularly.

So far, so good? There are innumerable ways for Maddie to begin her specific aims paragraph. You may come up with a better one. To this point she has described the problem in sufficient detail. Now she must summarize what is known about the specific problem (PF monitoring, not asthma in general), state what is not known (gap or gaps in knowledge), and end with the critical unmet need.

She continues,

> PF self-monitoring at home can be cumbersome for many children and families and, even with training, can be prone to poor technique and user error. Recording PF values regularly and knowing what to do when values drop can be challenging. There is a critical need to develop a system that encourages children and adolescents with asthma and their families to measure PF regularly and interpret and act upon the results before asthma symptoms worsen.

Maddie, as noted above, did test GuideFlow among a small sample of her patients. She may have obtained a small amount of pilot data, which can be described very briefly on the specific aims page and in more detail in the rest of the proposal. A sentence such as the following is sufficient:

> Among a small sample of 20 adolescent patients with asthma, all believed GuideFlow was easy to use and provided them with valuable information.

Maddie must now state the long-term goal of the proposed research and an overarching hypothesis. She continues,

> *Our long-term goal is to improve self-management of asthma among children and adolescents using a technology-based strategy to encourage regular PF monitoring and action based on PF values. Our overarching hypothesis is that a technology-based system is superior to routine PF monitoring education and monitoring using simple, currently widely available PF meters in preventing asthma morbidity and mortality.*

Notice that the purpose of each of the two sentences is absolutely clear with the inclusion of "Our long-term goal" and "Our overarching hypothesis."

Now let's consider the actual aims. These are often given a title that includes precisely what is to be accomplished, and each is accompanied by a hypothesis. Interdependency of aims should be avoided. For example, if the second aim relies upon the first being met successfully, this will depress enthusiasm for the proposal. Given space limitations, the aims must be succinct. Let's assume that Maddie is planning two aims. Don't worry about the precise mechanism of funding or other aspects that one would normally think about carefully in a grant application, and that would influence how the aims are formatted. Her first aim could be to carry out a randomized trial comparing GuideFlow to a more passive intervention. Her second aim could be to gain insights of the experience of patients with GuideFlow. Her first aim could be written as the following:

> Specific Aim #1: *To compare the GuideFlow system to asthma self-management education in a randomized trial among adolescents with asthma and at least one emergency room admission in the past 12 months.*

She packs a significant amount of information into this aim so that it describes what exactly will be compared and among whom. It wouldn't be appropriate to write more simply, "To compare GuideFlow to asthma self-management education in a randomized trial."

The aim should include a hypothesis, a guess or expectation of what Maddie hopes to find. It's already clear that she is interested in reducing asthma morbidity and mortality. These outcomes could be included in the aim as follows:

> *We hypothesize that patients in the GuideFlow arm of the trial will experience 25% fewer emergency room and hospital admissions than those in the asthma education (control) arm.*

It's best to be as specific as possible in stating the hypothesis. Maddie could have written only that GuideFlow would be associated with "significantly lower" admissions, but that might leave reviewers wondering what she meant by "significantly." Her hypothesis is relatively simple. She didn't include an expectation for a difference in asthma-related deaths. These are (fortunately) relatively rare and it would be hard to tell a difference between the two interventions.

Maddie's Specific Aim #1 is clearly very important and could form the basis of an entire research project itself. Few research proposals, however, have just one aim, and Maddie has additional questions she'd like to answer. Specifically, she is interested in the experience of patients with GuideFlow. She could collect this information from parents and children through interviews and analyze these qualitatively. This could be the foundation for a second aim:

Specific Aim #2: *To learn about the experience of patients and parents with the GuideFlow system through semi-structured telephone interviews.*

Notice again the specificity of the aim: She includes the mechanism through which the information is to be gathered. Like Specific Aim #1, #2 needs a hypothesis. Maddie anticipates that with its reminders, smartphone app, and automatic recording of values with accompanying advice, GuideFlow will be easy to use, especially among teens, who are often tech-savvy. Based on this hunch, she includes the following hypothesis:

We hypothesize that patients and parents will find GuideFlow easy to use, informative, and helpful overall in managing asthma.

There are no numbers, such as percentages, for this hypothesis since the aim relies on qualitative information.

Finally, let's consider the payoff or impact paragraph, which should summarize what is innovative about the proposal, what new knowledge will emerge, what impact the new knowledge will have, and how the proposal will advance the field. There is no precise formula for the impact paragraph. It must be short (three or four sentences).

Maddie could start with emphasizing the innovativeness of the proposal:

Our project will be the first to compare a technology-based system to encourage self-monitoring of PF in an adolescent population of asthma patients at high risk for asthma morbidity and mortality to routine asthma self-management education.

Next, she could summarize what new knowledge will emerge. This, of course, is available through the preceding paragraphs. Repetition for emphasis is helpful for building advocacy for the proposal. She could state:

We will measure the effectiveness of GuideFlow in preventing emergency room and hospital admissions, and also learn about the experience of patients with GuideFlow.

The impact of the new knowledge and advancement of the field could be captured in one sentence:

If successful, GuideFlow can be disseminated widely and inexpensively to children and adolescents with asthma, and an effective, technology-based solution to the challenge of self-monitoring of PF will advance the field of self-management of a common and serious chronic illness.

The example is simple, and the approach I've described above is just one among many that could have been taken. The challenge is writing a specific aims page clearly and persuasively. There are lots of variations, including those that place more emphasis on particular parts such as the background and impact paragraphs. Some discourage including citations in the specific aims page. I've included them in my own proposals and included the same citation numbers in other parts of the grant. To keep this example simple, let's leave them out.

Here's Maddie's completed specific aims page:

Too many poor children are hospitalized or die from asthma. In 2024, more than 700,000 children were admitted to emergency rooms or inpatient facilities with asthma exacerbations. There were more than 3,000 asthma-related deaths among children, a number that has been steadily increasing. Asthma self-management has been shown to reduce asthma exacerbations and therefore asthma-related morbidity and mortality. Regular peak-flow (PF) monitoring is an important, widely recommended component of asthma self-monitoring. Unfortunately, most children, including those at higher risk for asthma morbidity and mortality such as minority children and children from poor families, do not monitor PF regularly.

*PF self-monitoring at home can be cumbersome for many children and fam-
ilies and, even with training, can be prone to poor technique and user error.
Recording PF values regularly and knowing what to do when values drop can
be challenging. There is a critical need to develop a system that encourages
children and adolescents with asthma and their families to measure PF regularly and interpret and act upon the results before asthma symptoms worsen.
Among a small sample of 20 adolescent patients with asthma, all believed
GuideFlow was easy to use and provided them with valuable information.*

*Our long-term goal is to improve self-management of asthma among chil-
dren and adolescents using a technology-based strategy to encourage regular
PF monitoring and action based on PF values. Our overarching hypothesis is
that a technology-based system is superior to routine PF monitoring education
and monitoring using simple, widely available PF meters in preventing asthma
morbidity and mortality.*

Specific Aim #1*: To compare the GuideFlow system to asthma self-
management education in a randomized trial among adolescents with
asthma and at least one emergency room admission in the past 12 months.
We hypothesize that patients in the GuideFlow arm of the trial will experience
25% fewer emergency room and hospital admissions than those in the asthma
education (control) arm.*

Specific Aim #2*: To learn about the experience of patients and parents with the
GuideFlow system through semi-structured telephone interviews. We hypothesize that patients and parents will find GuideFlow easy to use, informative, and
helpful overall in managing asthma.*

*Our project will be the first to compare a technology-based system to en-
courage self-monitoring of PF in a pediatric population of asthma patients
at high risk for asthma morbidity and mortality to routine asthma self-
management education. We will measure the effectiveness of GuideFlow in
preventing emergency room and hospital admissions, and also about the experience of patients with GuideFlow. If successful, GuideFlow can be disseminated widely and inexpensively to children and adolescents with asthma, and
an effective, technology-based solution to the challenge of self-monitoring of
PF will advance the field of self-management of a common and serious chronic
illness.*

Table 9.1 summarizes, in general terms, how the 5Cs are applicable to the
specific aims page.

Table 9.1 The 5Cs and Specific Aims

Conciseness	Most grant funding agencies require the specific aims to be limited to one page or less. Conciseness, therefore, is absolutely necessary.
Cogency	The specific aims page needs to be persuasive to capture reviewers' attention and build advocacy for the proposal. Hence, Maddie's first sentence reads, "Too many poor children are hospitalized or die from asthma." Use the active voice whenever possible.
Clarity	Clarity is necessary for all scientific writing. Within the specific aims page, this is especially important when listing the actual aims. What is to be accomplished and what is hypothesized to happen must be 100% clear. Ask a colleague to read your actual aims to make sure he or she understands them the way you intended.
Commonness	Grant proposals are reviewed by diverse reviewers who may or may not have expertise in the subject matter of the proposal. Avoiding jargon is especially important in the specific aims page. A reviewer who doesn't know what an important term means may be less likely to advocate for the proposal. Whenever possible, define potentially unfamiliar jargon in your specific aims page rather than in other parts of the proposal so that reviewers have a good understanding of it before moving on.
Consistency	With some slight variations, the specific aims should follow the four-paragraph structure described above. Stick to it as closely as possible!

Specific Aims Exercise

You may already have a nice idea for a research project for which a specific aims page is needed. If so, go ahead and put it together. Here is a short exercise as well:

Guillermo is a hospitalist in a large academic health system. He has developed a strong interest in preventing readmissions among patients with exacerbations of chronic illnesses, congestive heart failure (CHF) in particular. He has seen too many of his patients with CHF be discharged after treatment for an exacerbation, only to return to the hospital within a week with worsening symptoms. To help solve the problem, Guillermo worked with a local home care agency and developed an innovative "CHF-Check In" program for patients recently discharged with CHF. Home care workers check in with recently discharged patients daily for 2 weeks by phone. Using a checklist Guillermo developed, they ask about symptoms, use of medications, change in body weight, and any other concerns the recently discharged patients might have. Phone checks are replaced by in-person visits if a patient is not doing well, or is unable or unwilling to answer the phone. Home care workers have contact information for relatives or friends of the patients to facilitate care and access to the home if needed. Guillermo's instinct is that the "CHF-Check In" is a good program that is having a significant impact on readmissions. The program is relatively inexpensive: Each home care worker looks after no more than 10 to 15 recently discharged patients, and contact is primarily by phone. He would like to evaluate the impact of the program formally by comparing it to usual care.

Construct the framework for a specific aims page that includes four sentences followed by statement of just one aim and a short sentence on impact. Don't worry about adding detail or references. The framework could form the basis for a more detailed specific aims page.

Suggested Response

Guillermo's opening sentence should describe the problem to be addressed and grab reviewers' attention. One possible opening is:

Many patients are discharged from the hospital for congestive heart failure (CHF) only to be readmitted soon afterwards.

Next, Guillermo can note what is known about the problem:

Poor self-care after discharge is a significant driver of readmission.

A sentence on the critical gap in knowledge comes next:

While home care services are widely available, it is unknown if a home care program to prevent CHF readmission is effective.

Finally, a sentence on the overarching goal of the proposed research is appropriate:

Our goal was to determine the effectiveness of a comprehensive home care program to prevent readmissions.

A potential single aim of the research is:

Specific Aim: *To determine if a home care program entitled "CHF-Check In" is effective compared to usual care in preventing readmissions from CHF.*

Notice the similarity between the final opening sentence and the aim. The aim provides more detail—nothing wrong with a bit of repetition for impact.

Guillermo could state his hypothesis as follows:

We hypothesize that compared with usual care, CHF-Check In will be associated with a 40% decrease in readmissions over a 12-month period.

A possible final impact statement is below:

Should CHF-Check In prove effective in reducing readmissions, it will represent an innovative approach to reducing overall CHF morbidity and mortality by taking advantage of existing home care services.

10

Grant Writing

Background and Significance

Though your grant proposal won't get very far if your specific aims are unsound, it can be argued that, overall, all three principal components of a grant application discussed in this book are equally important. You will not succeed if there are serious flaws in any of them. The specific aims are *what* you plan to accomplish. The approach section is *how* you plan to achieve your aims. The focus of this chapter is on *why* reviewers should consider your proposal. All granting bodies require the *why* in some form. The relevant sections in National Institutes of Health (NIH) proposals used to be called "background" and "significance." More recently, the required section has been changed to just "significance." The change in title is important because "background" implies a thorough review of what has been previously done, including the limitations of prior studies. "Significance," however, implies a rationale or an argument for the proposed research. While the recommended or required titles may vary among different granting bodies in different countries, what is expected is remarkably uniform. The Canadian Institutes of Health Research (CIHR), for example, require a brief "background and rationale."[1] The United Kingdom's Medical Research Council calls the equivalent section "importance."[2] For convenience, I will refer to this part of a grant proposal as "significance" from now on, following the NIH terminology.

Accompanying this section in NIH proposals is a brief section called "innovation" that we'll touch upon as well. "Innovation," "impact," or similar accompanying sections can be considered extensions of the significance section.

There are a few important principles to keep in mind as you prepare your significance section:

1. The significance section should not be an exhaustive review of prior research, technical details, or related information. Including too much

---

[1] https//www.queensu.ca/vpr/sites/vprwww/files/uploaded_files/Funding%20Sources/CIHR/CIHR-Project-Scheme-URS-Help-Files-Bundle.pdf. Accessed June 2, 2024.

[2] https://www.ukri.org/publications/mrc-guidance-for-applicants/. Accessed June 2, 2024.

detail is a common error in this section. Proposal reviewers have limited time. They are looking for a compelling rationale for the research, not a comprehensive education about the problem you are trying to address. You could argue that this section is necessarily limited in length given the required maximum length of the entire research proposal. However, you do have discretion within the maximum length (e.g., 12 pages, plus 1 page for specific aims for most NIH proposals). I would recommend you aim for no more than 1 to 2 pages.

2. The significance section should take the form of a carefully crafted argument for the proposed research. Imagine that you have 5 minutes to speak to an educated reviewer who knows almost nothing about the topic of your research. You need to convince him or her that the problem you wish to address is important, that prior solutions have failed or are suboptimal, that a significant gap in knowledge remains, that you have a strategy for addressing the gap, and that, by addressing the gap, our overall knowledge, clinical care, public health, etc. will be improved. Crafting this argument should be systematic, and we'll discuss a strategy for doing so.

3. The way you write the significance section is crucial. To keep reviewers engaged in your argument, use short, bold sentences. In other words, be concise and cogent. Divide this section into subheadings that follow a logical order or follow a consistent form. Make sure the meaning of each sentence is absolutely clear, and avoid jargon that may be unfamiliar to readers as much as possible. In other words, be conscious of all 5Cs as you write this section.

Scenario: *Rahul is a health services researcher who has observed, spoken about, and written about the devastating impact of lung cancer and the sub-optimal levels of lung cancer screening with low-dose computed tomography (LDCT) scanning among smokers and ex-smokers at risk. Through preliminary work, he has identified several reasons for poor screening rates: reluctance among patients to undergo LDCT screening, failure of physicians to order LDCT screening, and difficulty in identifying who is eligible for screening based on screening history. It is this last barrier that he wishes to address in a research project for which he wants to write a compelling significance section.*

Of course, the way in which you structure the significance section will depend greatly upon the topic, the granting body to which you are applying, and where you wish to place emphasis in your application. While there is no single formula, taking a careful look at the strategy and content I describe should help you understand the principles listed above and apply them to other significance sections.

There is a large amount of advice available online and elsewhere on how to write a significance section for NIH proposals. The advice is largely uniform and also consistent with the advice provided by other granting bodies in the United States and governmental and other bodies in other countries. Rather than reviewing all this advice, I recommend two key resources to use before you start writing your section:

1. Read sample significance sections for successful grant applications (e.g., https://www.niaid.nih.gov/grants-contracts/sample-applications).
2. Review the explicit criteria that NIH study sections use for peer review of proposals, including the following criteria for evaluating significance:
   a. Does the project address an important problem or a critical barrier to progress in the field?
   b. If the aims of the project are achieved, how will scientific knowledge, technical capability, and/or clinical practice be improved?
   c. How will successful completion of the aims change the concepts, methods, technologies, treatments, services, or preventative interventions that drive this field?

Keep these three questions close by as you write your significance section, and, once you've completed it, be sure you've answered all three. Though valuable in writing a significance section that meets NIH requirements, I've always found these questions a bit ambiguous and redundant. For example, "successful completion of the aims" for "improving technical capability" seems awfully similar to "completion of the aims" for changing "technologies." As you review your draft significance section, you might find you have the same response to parts of different questions. There's nothing wrong with that. Just as there is some redundancy built into the review criteria, I also advise you to be repetitive at times. Hammer home the significance by highlighting aspects of your rationale for the project several times, just to make sure reviewers get the message.

Now let's get started with Rahul's scenario.

He should structure his significance section in short paragraphs, each beginning with a sentence that is bold in style but also in typeface! Each short paragraph should represent a step in the rationale. By the time reviewers get to the end, there should be no doubt as to why the project is important. He should start broadly with a description of the problem of lung cancer. Since this section includes background information that needs to be substantiated with citations, it is especially dense with citations. Since this is a book about writing and not the quality or quantity of evidence for specific statements, I've limited the number of citations in the sample. You should, by contrast, substantiate each short paragraph with as many citations as you feel are needed.

Rahul could start with something like:

Recent epidemiological studies report an annual incidence of lung cancer in the United States of . . .

But that wouldn't be very cogent. There are better ways to get reviewers' attention. Here is a sample first short paragraph:

Too many Americans die from lung cancer. *In 2024, there were an estimated 234,580 cases of lung cancer in the United States, resulting in 125,070 deaths.*[3]

Two short sentences are fine for an opening paragraph. Rahul may want to point out that lung cancer disproportionately affects certain groups, etc. in the same paragraph, depending upon the focus of his proposed study.

Now that he's summarized the problem, the next step would be to discuss the value of LDCT screening for early detection of lung cancer. This paragraph should begin with what seems obvious, that early detection of lung cancer saves lives. Remember that the section should take the form of a logical, stepwise argument for the research. It's always best not to skip a step or make assumptions about what reviewers might already know:

Early detection of lung cancer saves lives. *Scanning with low-dose computed tomography (LDCT) is a safe and accurate way to detect lung cancer early.*[4]

These two short sentences are succinct and cogent. Rahul may wish to embellish the short paragraph with additional details about the number of lives that can be saved through LDCT screening. Notice the simple, bold language in the first sentence. "Early detection . . . saves lives" catches reviewers' attention better than "Early detection . . . improves survival," for example.

As a next step, Rahul may wish to point out that in addition to the benefits of LDCT screening observed in research studies, screening through this method

[3] Siegel RL, Giaquinto AN, Jemal A. Cancer statistics, 2024. *CA Cancer J Clin* 2024;74(1):12–49.
[4] Henschke CI, Yip R, Shaham, D, et al. A 20-year follow-up of the International Early Lung Cancer Action Program (I-ELCAP). Radiology 2023;309(2):e231988. doi:10.1148/radiol.231988

is recommended by authoritative organizations. Rahul needs to make it even more clear that LDCT screening should be taking place. It is simply another stepping stone in his argument:

> **LDCT is a recommended screening procedure.** *The U.S. Preventive Services Task Force (USPSTF) recommends annual screening for lung cancer with LDCT in adults aged 50 to 80 who have a 20 pack-year history of smoking and currently smoke or have quit within the past 15 years.*[5]

You might wonder if the first sentence in this short paragraph is truly necessarily; wouldn't it be more concise to begin with "The U.S. Preventive Services Task Force"? However, by stating that LDCT screening is recommended, it continues to build the argument in a stepwise fashion. Simply stating the USPSTF recommendation makes it harder for reviewers to recognize the next step in the argument.

Now it's time for Rahul to describe the main problem he wishes to address. While lung cancer is deadly and a tool for early detection is both available and recommended, screening rates are low:

> **Unfortunately, screening rates are abysmal.** *The 2022 State of Lung Cancer report from the American Lung Association revealed that just 5.8% of eligible Americans receive LDCT screening.*[6]

Again, the two sentences complement each other. The first makes a bold, cogent point. The second substantiates it. Rahul could add additional evidence for low rates of screening. This would be perfectly reasonable given how short his section is so far.

Reviewers should be able to follow his logic to this point, and the next question they might wonder about is the "why" of low screening rates. Rahul could continue:

> **Low screening rates are the result of many factors.**[7] *There are patient factors such as a lack of interest in screening and mistrust of the medical system.*

---

[5] https://www.uspreventiveservicestaskforce.org/uspstf/recommendation/lung-cancer-screening. Accessed June 4, 2024.

[6] https://www.lung.org/getmedia/647c433b-4cbc-4be6-9312-2fa9a449d489/solc-2022-print-report. Accessed June 4, 2024.

[7] Cavers D, Nelson M, Rostron J, et al. Understanding patient barriers and facilitators to uptake of lung screening using low dose computed tomography: A mixed methods scoping review of the current literature. Respir Res 2022;23:374. https://doi.org/10.1186/s12931-022-02255-8

System factors include a lack of access to screening. Physician factors include a lack of knowledge about screening guidelines and a lack of information about eligibility of individual patients. It is this last barrier that is the focus of our proposal.

Rahul provided a general summary of barriers. He could expand by providing more details about the barriers, but he should avoid a comprehensive summary of literature on this topic. Notice that his last sentence is not background information. It could also appear in the aims of the proposal. Redundancy here and there to hammer home the point to reviewers, as mentioned above, is perfectly acceptable.

At this point, reviewers might be curious about what he means by "lack of information about eligibility." He should explain this in his next paragraph clearly and concisely.

It's too cumbersome with current electronic health record (EHR) tools to identify which patients are eligible for screening due to inaccurate or incomplete smoking histories. Kuchareva and colleagues describe inaccuracy in smoking history data as a major barrier to identifying eligibility for LDCT screening and higher screening rates.[8]

Notice the pattern of a cogent sentence backed up by evidence.

The last step is for Rahul to describe a potential solution, not necessarily his specific solution, but an idea for how to solve the problem. Backing up the idea with evidence for a similar intervention is always wise:

A simple, discrete tool consisting of short questions that patients complete in advance of an appointment could help identify screening eligibility and also provide patients with information about the value of screening. "Pre-visit planning tools" have been used successfully to improve patient empowerment and delivery of care and could be helpful in improving the accuracy and completeness of smoking histories.[9]

---

[8] Kukhareva PV, Caverly TJ, Li H, et al. Inaccuracies in electronic health records smoking data and a potential approach to address resulting underestimation in determining lung cancer screening eligibility. J Am Med Inform Assoc 2022 Apr 13;29(5):779–788. doi:10.1093/jamia/ocac020. PMID: 35167675; PMCID: PMC9006678.

[9] Gholamzadeh M, Abtahi H, Ghazisaeeidi M. Applied techniques for putting pre-visit planning in clinical practice to empower patient-centered care in the pandemic era: A systematic review and framework suggestion. BMC Health Serv Res 2021;21(1):458. doi:10.1186/s12913-021-06456-7. PMID: 33985502; PMCID: PMC8116646.

The logic in Rahul's section is sound: Lung cancer is a big problem → Early detection saves lives → LDCT screening is accurate and safe → LDCT screening is underused → Inaccurate/incomplete smoking history is a barrier to use → Pre-visit tools could help with improving smoking histories.

This example is very simple and doesn't include a lot of substantiating data and citations. When the logic is more complex or the evidence you wish to include in your significance section is more exhaustive, it's a good idea to start with a few basic sentences connected by arrows, such as what I did above, to provide an outline for the section and to make sure your logic is sound.

Accompanying the significance section in NIH proposals is a section on innovation. Some granting bodies may require describing innovation and overall impact as part of a single section, titled "background" for example. Here are the NIH's specific instructions for reviews to evaluate the innovativeness of a proposal:[10]

- Evaluate the extent to which innovation influences the importance of undertaking the proposed research. Note that while technical or conceptual innovation can influence the importance of the proposed research, a project that is not applying novel concepts or approaches may be of critical importance for the field.
- Evaluate whether the proposed work applies novel concepts, methods or technologies or uses existing concepts, methods, technologies in novel ways, to enhance the overall impact of the project.

Essentially, Rahul needs to convey in one short paragraph what is innovative about his proposed research and why its innovativeness will have a significant impact. The first bullet point asks reviewers to assess innovation as a driver of the research but points out that even if there are no new concepts or approaches, the research might still be important. Consider the application of an existing tool, treatment, etc. to a completely new population (e.g., adults versus children). The second bullet point explicitly asks reviewers not *if* there is innovation, but what specifically is innovative.

Innovation is best summarized in a short, bulleted paragraph. Three or four bullets are customary. Here is how Rahul could describe innovation:

- *Our approach is to extend the well-established strategy of pre-visit tools to enhance patient engagement and quality of care to acquiring smoking history data for the purpose of determining eligibility for LDCT screening.*

---

[10] https://grants.nih.gov/policy/peer/simplifying–review/framework.htm. Accessed June 5, 2024.

Notice that Rahul describes an existing strategy. He's not describing a completely novel method for gathering information for patients. He plans to merely extend an existing one to a new and important problem.

- *Our study will be the first to apply pre-visit smoking questionnaires for the purpose of lung cancer screening.*

This is a novel application of a tool.

- *Our study tackles a significant barrier to lung cancer screening—identifying which patients are eligible. The screening questionnaire will be accompanied by information about LDCT screening for patients to review. Ours will be the first study to empower patients with knowledge about their own eligibility for screening and about the screening process.*

The empowerment of patients for lung cancer screening is described as innovative.

- *If our aims are met, we expect more discussions of lung cancer screening between physicians and patients and substantially higher screening rates, leading to higher rates of early detection of lung cancer, and lower morbidity and mortality.*

This last point doesn't describe innovation, but rather the overall potential impact of the research. This could be placed elsewhere or repeated in different forms in the aims or significance sections. As noted, there is nothing wrong with being a bit repetitive to hammer the point home.

Table 10.1 describes the application of the 5Cs to the significance section.

Significance Exercise

Gestational diabetes is a serious problem associated with worse pregnancy and birth outcomes and affects many women in the United Kingdom and many other highly developed countries. In 2020, Laura Kusinski and her colleagues published an article in the journal *Nutrients* describing a protocol for a study of a dietary intervention among women with gestational diabetes to mitigate both maternal weight gain during pregnancy and infant birthweight.[11] Your

---

[11] Kusinski LC, Murphy HR, De Lucia Rolfe E, et al. Dietary intervention in pregnant women with gestational diabetes; protocol for the DiGest randomised controlled trial. Nutrients 2020 Apr

Table 10.1 5Cs and Significance

Conciseness	Use short sentences that are easy to follow. A short significance section gives you more room for the approach section of your proposal. Keep in mind you can point out the significance of your proposed work a few times in different places. Don't provide exhaustive reviews or background information. Reviewers will find that tedious, and the all-important logic underlying your proposal may be lost.
Cogency	Your sentences should be short, bold, and direct. Use bold-faced font to begin each short paragraph.
Clarity	Make sure the logic in your significance section is clear. It's helpful to write down a few phrases before writing the entire section and to make sure they are connected in a logical, stepwise fashion.
Commonness	It's crucial to avoid jargon that reviewers may not understand in this section. Reviewers should be able to read this section quickly and easily to follow your logic. You don't want them looking up terms or concepts and thereby disrupting the process through which they understand the importance of your proposed research.
Consistency	Follow the form for the significance section described above. It's useful as a logical framework and it's also what reviewers are accustomed to reading.

task is to read the following introduction to the study and to construct no more than six short sentences that could form the basic framework for a significance section, and no more than two additional sentences that describe innovation. Don't worry about citations.

Gestational diabetes (GDM) affects around 5% of pregnant women in the United Kingdom (UK) [1] and increases the risk of suboptimal materno-fetal outcomes and is associated with pre-pregnancy obesity and excessive gestational weight gain [2–5]. GDM is usually diagnosed at 24–28 weeks' gestation and identifies women at risk of type 2 diabetes in later life. Although excessive gestational weight gain in early pregnancy (0–28 weeks) is well-established as a risk factor for GDM [3], the role of weight control in women after the diagnosis of GDM, from 28 weeks to delivery, is unclear.

Weight gain is a normal part of a healthy pregnancy, but excessive weight gain can contribute to poor outcomes for both the mother and child. Excessive gestational weight gain is currently defined using the Institute of Medicine guidelines (2009) based upon a woman's pre-pregnancy body mass index (BMI) [6]. Normal weight, overweight, and obese women are advised to gain 11.4–15.9 kg, 6.8–11.4 kg, and 5.0–9.1 kg, respectively [6]. Many pregnant women exceed these targets and gain excessive weight [7]. It is also unclear if these

22;12(4):1165. doi:10.3390/nu12041165. Erratum in: Nutrients 2020;12(6):1793. doi:10.3390/nu12061793. PMID: 32331244; PMCID: PMC7230897.

targets are suitable for women with GDM, who are already at higher risk of ad-verse pregnancy outcomes compared with women without diabetes [5] and who may benefit from lower gestational weight gain targets [8]. It is unclear if maternal weight gain after GDM diagnosis remains important to prevent ad-verse maternal and baby outcomes, but there are data that suggest this is the case. A study by Harper and colleagues showed that for every 1 lb per week increase in weight in women after diagnosis with GDM, there was a 36–83% increased risk for pre-eclampsia, caesarean section, macrosomia, and large-for-gestational-age (LGA) (7). The guidelines of the National Institute of Health and Care Excellence (NICE) for diabetes in pregnancy highlight the importance of pre-pregnancy and post-partum weight control in women with GDM, but do not provide guidance on gestational weight gain targets [9]. There is currently limited evidence to guide clinical practice in this area.

Excessive weight gain has been associated with multiple adverse outcomes. In the general obstetric population, excessive gestational weight gain has been associated with hypertensive disorders in pregnancy [10], LGA [11], macrosomia [12], depression [13], and may also be linked to infant death [14]. In later life, women with excessive gestational weight gain during pregnancy are at increased risk of type 2 diabetes and cardiometabolic disease [15], which may be linked to the weight gained in pregnancy not being completely lost after the birth [16]. Offspring of women with excessive gestational weight gain have increased body weight, increased fat mass, and increased blood pressure in childhood, raising concerns about obesity and diabetes risk in later life [17–19].

Women with GDM and who are overweight or obese pre-pregnancy may benefit from minimal gestational weight gain in later pregnancy to improve both short- and longer-term health outcomes. Theoretically, reduced late gestational weight gain may improve infant birth weight and impact upon postpartum weight retention and future cardiometabolic risk. However, few studies have ever assessed pregnancy outcomes following moderate energy restriction in women with GDM [20,21]. These studies have been useful in pro-viding evidence for maternal and neonatal outcomes, however they did not provide comprehensive evidence that having a strict food allocation over a set period of time could impact on these outcomes, as addressed in this protocol.

The clinical trial protocol presented here is a double-blind, fully controlled dietary intervention using a novel approach of diet boxes. Diet boxes have be-come very popular commercially and contain all of an individual's meals and snacks for the week delivered to their home or workplace. Meals are designed to be nutritionally balanced, healthy, appetising and require only minimal time and effort to cook at home. As participants can be randomised to receive a box providing reduced or standard energy diet, this overcomes many of the challenges faced in controlling and blinding nutritional studies in free-living pregnant volunteers.

The aim of this trial is to identify if a reduced energy diet in 500 pregnant women diagnosed with GDM can reduce gestational weight gain, improve pregnancy outcomes, and reduce postnatal glucose concentrations.

Suggested Response

There are many ways to build a logical framework that explains the significance of the study. As in the example of Rahul's study above, you should start with a description of the problem and its seriousness. Here's one possible set of six sentences for significance:

1. *Gestational diabetes (GDM) is a common and serious problem associated with maternal and infant complications.* →
2. *There is a clear relationship between pregnancy weight gain and GDM, as excessive weight gain is a risk factor for GDM.* →
3. *There are guidelines for weight gain in normal pregnancies.* →
4. *However, levels of weight gain lower than those recommended in normal pregnancies have been associated with better outcomes in women with GDM.*
5. *It is also known that energy restriction in women with GDM can improve outcomes.*
6. *It is unknown, however, if strict food allocation over an extended period of time in pregnancy is associated with better outcomes in women with GDM.*

The logic should be clear. You might consider sentence number 2 unnecessary; after all, the study is not about risk factors for GDM, but rather how to manage patients who already have GDM. I suggested it, though, because it points out what we already know about GDM and weight gain. Some reviewers might not be aware of this relationship, and jumping from the seriousness of gestational diabetes to guidelines for weight gain and the benefits of lower weight gain among women with GDM might confuse reviewers who aren't aware that weight and GDM are related.

Here are a couple of suggestions for innovation:

1. *A few studies have shown that energy restriction in GDM leads to improved outcomes.*
2. *Our study will be the first to extend energy restriction for a longer duration in pregnancy and to evaluate its impact in a randomized trial.*

The first sentence makes it clear that the idea of energy restriction is not entirely novel. The second sentence describes precisely what *is* novel.

11
Grant Writing
Approach

The specific aims section of your proposal is *what* you plan to do. The significance section is *why* you plan to do it. The approach section is *how* you plan to do it. All three of these sections, of course, are critically important. After reading the specific aims and significance, reviewers should come to an understanding of the importance of your research. The approach section is the longest of these three sections and includes lots of details. In this section, reviewers are less concerned with understanding the overall importance of your research and more concerned about the soundness of your methodology. As with all the other chapters in this book, what goes in the approach section will vary tremendously depending upon the subject matter, funding opportunity, and grant sponsoring organization. Also, this chapter will not help make sure your approach is methodologically sound. But it should help you convey your methodology clearly and concisely so that reviewers are better able to judge the soundness of your idea. As with other sections of a proposal, there are a few important principles to keep in mind:

1. The fifth of the 5Cs, *consistency*, is essential to adhere to in writing your approach section. This section is typically dense, with many technical details. You should make it as easy to follow as possible for reviewers. A useful way to do this is to divide your approach into sections for each aim, and to further divide these into subsections. These should be lettered or numbered in sequence. This type of organization makes it easier for reviewers to get around. For example, as you write a paragraph in one subsection, you can state, for example, "See also C.6 for additional details." Reviewers who have questions about what you've written can immediately find "C.6" and hopefully find answers. Without well-organized sections and subsections, your approach may resemble a jumbled mess, and reviewers will struggle to make their way through it.

2. In general, every part of the approach section should be linked to the specific aims. Organizing the approach with sections for each aim will

help in this regard, but don't include methods, or procedures that fall outside of the aims. For example, in a proposal that is designed to evaluate pulmonary function and hospitalizations as primary outcomes, you may wish to carry out a survey of satisfaction of participants in a pulmonary rehabilitation program. You shouldn't just throw the survey into the approach, for it will seem out of place. Instead, include it as an aim, or part of an aim, as a plan to assess the satisfaction of participants with the rehabilitation program. The National Institutes of Health (NIH) and other granting sections often require or recommend a section on "preliminary studies" or prior work you have completed that supports the current proposal. Even this section should be linked to the aims. You should make it clear how your prior work provides a foundation for one or more aims.

3. Anticipate concerns or questions as you write your approach. This will make your proposal cogent and authoritative. For example, say you are using an older assay instrument in part of a study and are aware that newer instruments are available. You should include at some point something to the effect of, "We acknowledge that the instrument we plan to use has largely been replaced. However, some of our sites do not have access to the newer instrument, and we have decided to use the older instrument for uniformity of measurement technique and standards." In NIH and other proposals, anticipated concerns are often included as a separate section entitled "Challenges and Limitations" in which you can summarize concerns and provide detailed responses. Imagine you are a reviewer with some familiarity with the methodology in your approach section. A nagging problem that has confronted you in your research or some of your colleagues' research immediately comes to mind as you read a paragraph in the approach. Imagine that your confidence in the success of the proposal would increase substantially if you find a cogent response to the concern soon after reading the paragraph. The likelihood of the proposal being rated favorably would also increase.

4. A picture is worth a thousand words, and this idea certainly applies to your approach section: Use "pictures" whenever possible. Graphs, charts, and figures serve two key purposes. First, they allow you to convey a large amount of information in limited space. Space is always limited in your approach section and your overall research strategy. Second, they provide a guide or useful summary for key parts of the section. Imagine that you have a detailed stepwise strategy for how you plan to identify and recruit patients for a study. It may start with a query of a particular database of patients and proceed with contacting eligible participants, etc. If the flow of patients through your study is complex,

describing the flow in a single, dense paragraph within the approach section would turn off reviewers. Instead, it's better to summarize the flow in a couple of sentences, and then include a figure with additional details, which makes it easier for reviewers to follow.

Let's extend Rahul's scenario in Chapter 10 to encompass his approach section. As you may recall, Rahul is interested in improving uptake of low-dose computed tomography (LDCT) screening for early detection of lung cancer. He has identified inaccurate and/or incomplete smoking histories as a significant barrier. Let's assume he has three relatively straightforward aims:

Specific Aim #1: *In collaboration with primary care physicians and patients, develop and refine an accurate and practical tool for gathering smoking history information from patients who have ever smoked.*

We hypothesize that a simple questionnaire tool can be developed that provides accurate smoking history information and which can be completed by patients in less than five minutes.

Specific Aim #2: *Include the tool in pre-visit questionnaires sent to adult patients in advance of annual checkup visits, and make completed questionnaire information available to physicians in electronic health records.*

We hypothesize that the majority (60%) of adult patients who have ever smoked presenting for annual checkup visits will complete the questionnaire on their mobile phones.

Specific Aim #3: *Measure the impact of the tool in a cluster-randomized trial of primary care practices within a large, integrated primary care network.*

We hypothesize that compared to usual care, in which only 10% of eligible patients receive LDCT, 40% of eligible patients in practices in which the tool has been deployed will receive LDCT.

Rahul plans to submit his proposal to the NIH, which provides the following instructions for the approach section:

1. Describe the overall strategy, methodology, and analyses to be used to accomplish the specific aims of the project.
2. Describe the experimental design and methods proposed and how they will achieve robust and unbiased results.
3. Unless addressed separately in the Resource Sharing Plan, include how the data will be collected, analyzed, and interpreted as well as any resource sharing plans as appropriate.

4. For trials that randomize groups or deliver interventions to groups, describe how your methods for analysis and sample size are appropriate for your plans for participant assignment and intervention delivery. These methods can include a group- or cluster-randomized trial or an individually randomized group-treatment trial.

5. Discuss potential problems, alternative strategies, and benchmarks for success anticipated to achieve the aims.

6. If the project is in the early stages of development, describe any strategy to establish feasibility, and address the management of any high-risk aspects of the proposed work.

7. Explain how relevant biological variables, such as sex, are factored into research designs and analyses for studies in vertebrate animals and humans. For example, strong justification from the scientific literature, preliminary data, or other relevant considerations must be provided for applications proposing to study only one sex.

8. Point out any procedures, situations, or materials that may be hazardous to personnel and the precautions to be exercised.

There are additional instructions as well, but these are the principal ones we'll consider when applicable to Rahul's scenario. These instructions might seem obvious, and may be sections Rahul had already planned to include, but I believe they are useful in organizing the approach. In fact, using some of the language for "headings" in the approach, such as "overall strategy," will convince reviewers that the proposal has been designed to meet the funder's requirements.

Now, Rahul can move on to an organizational framework. The key portions of a grant proposal, namely the aims, significance, and approach, are organized in many successful proposals into lettered headings—A for the aims, B, for significance, and C for approach. Subheadings such as C.1, C.2, etc. help keep the approach section organized and easy to follow. For the NIH and other funding bodies, there is no precise, prescriptive way to do this. However, a common framework I've used in health services research applications is:

C.1 *Overall strategy*: A summary of all the research procedures. It's fine to start with the overall purpose of the study. This should be a single paragraph that provides a useful foundation for the more detailed description of the research procedures that follows.

C.2 *Preliminary studies*: Prior work that supports the need for or provides a foundation for the proposed research. As noted, this prior work should be directly related to the aims of the proposal.

C.3 *Research procedures for the first aim*: I would repeat the first aim here (without any hypotheses, to save space) and describe different elements of the first aim with additional subheadings (e.g., C.3.1, C.3.2). Alternatively, C.3 could be an overview of the setting or environment for the study, with the first aim beginning with C.4.

C.4 and C.5 *Research procedures for the second and third aims*, with additional subheadings as needed.

      C.6 *Sample size, power, and statistical analyses*: The primary and secondary outcomes for the study should be obvious throughout the proposal. There's nothing wrong with describing them in the aims, again in the "overall strategy" and research procedures for each aim, and again (briefly) in this subsection.

      C.7 *Challenges and alternative strategies*: In this section, anticipated challenges (which reviewers may also think about) should be addressed, along with ways to overcome them. These can also be described under each aim.

We'll focus on these seven sections, but additional sections may follow, including plans for dissemination (e.g., publication in journals), a timeline, etc.

Keep in mind that the approach section is all about detail. The aims and significance are intended to persuade reviewers that what you would like to do is important. The "science" portion of typical NIH proposals is 13 pages long (including the aims page). The approach section typically takes up 10 pages. Rather than providing Rahul's entire approach (which would make this chapter unnecessarily lengthy), below is a detailed description and key features of what might go into each of the seven sections above, with a scheme for further subheadings:

C.1 *Overall strategy*: It's reasonable for Rahul to summarize, once again, the purpose of the study, along with a capsule summary of the aims, in two opening sentences, such as:

> *Our goal is to address the lack of an accurate and complete smoking history as a barrier to identifying patients eligible for LDCT. We will develop and implement a simple pre-visit tool for completion by patients to obtain accurate smoking histories and measure the impact of the tool on screening rates in a cluster-randomized trial.*

C.2 *Preliminary studies*: Preliminary studies can take many forms. They can be smaller versions of what is being proposed for a larger study. They can also provide valuable foundational work for the proposal.

They can provide additional evidence for the need for the study. Let's say Rahul has surveyed a large number of physicians who report that difficulty in obtaining an accurate smoking history is a barrier to LDCT screening. He would include details of the survey in this section. The section could begin with:

> C.2 *Preliminary Study: Survey of primary care physicians on barriers to LDCT screening. We surveyed 130 primary care physicians about barriers to LDCT screening. A lack of knowledge of screening guidelines and the difficulty in obtaining accurate smoking histories were cited as the most significant barriers . . .*

C.3 *Research procedures for the first aim*: Rahul should start by restating the aim in bold font:

> C.3 **Specific Aim #1**: *In collaboration with primary care physicians and patients, develop and refine an accurate and practical tool for gathering smoking history information.*

A useful next step is to make an outline of each of the procedures for the aim by listing the steps that will be taken. Each step can be specified with a numbered subheading. Here's one scheme:

> C.3.1 *Panel of physician and patients*: Rahul could describe the recruitment and composition of a small panel of physicians and patients who will participate in this aim.
>
> C.3.2 *Presentation of a draft tool*: Rahul could state that a draft tool developed by the research team will be presented to the panel, who will then be asked for feedback about clarity, usefulness, etc. (More details can be included, such as taking notes and analyzing these afterwards.) The tool will be refined based on feedback.
>
> C.3.3 *Testing of tool*: Rahul could describe testing of the tool among a small sample of patients (20 to 30) for ease of completion and additional feedback, based on which additional refinements could be made.

Notice that each subheading describes a specific step in fulfilling the aim. Here's a comparable outline for the second and third aims:

C.4 **Specific Aim #2**: *Include the tool in pre-visit questionnaires sent to adult patients in advance of annual checkup visits and make completed questionnaire information available to physicians in electronic health records.*

C.4.1 *Technical development—incorporating questionnaire*: Rahul could describe the technical procedures for incorporating the pre-visit questionnaire into existing communication tools for patients, such as an electronic health records portal, text messaging etc. This sub-aim could include refinement of the format and appearance of the questionnaire based on patient feedback.

C.4.2 *Technical development—physician interface*: Rahul could describe the technical procedures for incorporating questionnaire results into the physician view of the patient's electronic health record. This sub-aim could include refinement of the format and appearance of the physician interface based on physicians' feedback.

C.5 **Specific Aim #3**: *Measure the impact of the tool in a cluster-randomized trial of primary care practices within a large, integrated primary care network.*

C.5.1 *Practice network overview*: Rahul could describe the network of practices, including its size, geographic distribution, and physician/provider and patient population characteristics.

C.5.2 *Design of cluster-randomized trial*: As practices, as opposed to patients, will be randomized to the questionnaire intervention or usual care (or another type of intervention), Rahul could describe the randomization procedures, including how practices will be balanced in each arm based on size, characteristics, etc.

C.5.3 *Rollout of interventions*: Rahul could describe the rollout of the questionnaire in the intervention arm, including the timing of requests for questionnaire completion with respect to annual wellness visits, etc. The control arm could receive usual care with no inclusion of any lung cancer screening effort. Alternatively, patients could receive general information on LDCT through the same communication channels describe for Specific Aim #2. A flow diagram is useful in describing the path of patients in each arm through the study.

C.5.4 *Outcomes to be measured*: Rahul could describe the primary and secondary outcomes he is most interested in, along with how they will be measured. These could include questionnaire completion rates, LDCT scans completed (screening rate), and even detection of lung cancer. He could also measure satisfaction among physicians/providers and patients with the questionnaires. Note that if he plans to measure satisfaction, this outcome should be included in the specific aims.

C.6 *Sample size, power, and statistical analyses*: This section should be as detailed as possible, and Rahul should provide a reasonable calculation that supports the anticipated sample of patients who will participate in the program as adequate to demonstrate a significant difference between intervention and control arms. The statistical analyses to be completed to measure the outcomes listed in C.5.4 should be described in detail, including the planned statistical procedures and any software to be used.

C.7 *Challenges and alternative strategies*: This section is an excellent opportunity for Rahul to anticipate concerns about the study among reviewers and to demonstrate that he not only is aware of these concerns but also has a strategy to address them. For example, some practices in the practice network may refuse to participate. If this happens, Rahul can describe how a second network of practices can provide alternative sites for the study.

Though what we've described here is a general outline of Rahul's approach section, keep in mind that he should include as much detail as possible. The flow of his study is relatively straightforward, so I've suggested only one diagram to describe participant flow. Other studies could benefit from more than one diagram, chart, or table for greater clarity.

Table 11.1 describes the application of the 5Cs to the approach section of a research proposal.

Approach Exercise

Dementia is a devastating condition, and its prevalence is increasing rapidly as the global population ages.[1] Effective treatments are elusive, and even slowing

[1] GBD 2019 Dementia Forecasting Collaborators. Estimation of the global prevalence of dementia in 2019 and forecasted prevalence in 2050: An analysis for the Global Burden of Disease Study 2019. Lancet Public Health 2022 Feb;7(2):e105–e125. doi:10.1016/S2468-2667(21)00249-8. Epub 2022 Jan 6. PMID: 34998485; PMCID: PMC8810394.

Table 11.1 5Cs and Approach

Conciseness	As in all scientific writing, use short sentences that are easy to follow. The content under each subheading should be concise. Don't hesitate to break up initially longer sections into two with separate subheadings. Given the amount of detail in the approach section, short subsections are easier to follow than longer ones.
Cogency	Use the active voice and put statements in positive form, as always—for instance, "We will recruit practices from across the network" versus "Practices from across the network will be recruited."
Clarity	The logical flow of your approach will depend to a great extent on how it's organized, but make sure each subsection is absolutely clear and related to the ones that precede and follow it. Always make sure each subsection is closely related to the aims of your study.
Commonness	Using jargon is unavoidable for the approach section, but make sure you define terms that may be unfamiliar to reviewers. Spell out any abbreviations the first time they are used, even if they are commonly used in your field.
Consistency	Consistency is of critical importance. Organize your approach in sections and subheadings as described above. A dense page that is not split into sections will immediately turn off reviewers.

down the progression of various forms of dementia such as Alzheimer disease has proven challenging. Measures to prevent dementia have received considerable attention in recent years. These include exercise, improved nutrition, effective treatment of hypertension, and others. Vaccines, including vaccines to prevent herpes zoster (shingles), have also shown some promise. Shingles vaccination is routinely recommended for adults aged 50 and older, and lower rates of dementia among those who receive the vaccine have been observed in several studies. However, it's possible that those who request and receive the vaccine are fundamentally different from those who don't in ways that are related to the risk for dementia. For example, those who receive the vaccine might be more health conscious than others and may exercise more.

Your first task is to read this abstract from a paper by Eyting et al.:[2]

The root causes of dementia are still largely unclear, and the medical community lacks highly effective preventive and therapeutic pharmaceutical agents for dementia despite large investments into their development. There is growing interest in the question if infectious agents play a role in the development of dementia, with herpesviruses attracting particular attention. To

[2] Eyting M, Xie M, Heß S, Geldsetzer P. Causal evidence that herpes zoster vaccination prevents a proportion of dementia cases. medRxiv [Preprint]. May 25, 2023. doi:10.1101/2023.05.23.23290253. PMID: 37282746; PMCID: PMC10246135.

provide causal as opposed to merely correlational evidence on this question, we take advantage of the fact that in Wales eligibility for the herpes zoster vaccine (Zostavax) for shingles prevention was determined based on an individual's exact date of birth. Those born before September 2 1933 were ineligible and remained ineligible for life, while those born on or after September 2 1933 were eligible to receive the vaccine. By using country-wide data on all vaccinations received, primary and secondary care encounters, death certificates, and patients' date of birth in weeks, we first show that the percentage of adults who received the vaccine increased from 0.01% among patients who were merely one week too old to be eligible, to 47.2% among those who were just one week younger. Apart from this large difference in the probability of ever receiving the herpes zoster vaccine, there is no plausible reason why those born just one week prior to September 2 1933 should differ systematically from those born one week later. We demonstrate this empirically by showing that there were no systematic differences (e.g., in pre-existing conditions or uptake of other pre-ventive interventions) between adults across the date-of-birth eligibility cutoff, and that there were no other interventions that used the exact same date-of-birth eligibility cutoff as was used for the herpes zoster vaccine program. This unique natural randomization, thus, allows for robust causal, rather than correlational, effect estimation. We first replicate the vaccine's known effect from clinical trials of reducing the occurrence of shingles. We then show that receiving the herpes zoster vaccine reduced the probability of a new dementia diagnosis over a follow-up period of seven years by 3.5 percentage points (95% CI: 0.6–7.1, p = 0.019), corresponding to a 19.9% relative reduction in the oc-currence of dementia. Besides preventing shingles and dementia, the herpes zoster vaccine had no effects on any other common causes of morbidity and mortality. In exploratory analyses, we find that the protective effects from the vaccine for dementia are far stronger among women than men. Randomized trials are needed to determine the optimal population groups and time in-terval for administration of the herpes zoster vaccine to prevent or delay de-mentia, as well as to quantify the magnitude of the causal effect when more precise measures of cognition are used. Our findings strongly suggest an im-portant role of the varicella zoster virus in the etiology of dementia.

Fascinating, isn't it?

Now imagine that you have the opportunity to carry out a study along sim-ilar lines. In 2013 a large network of assisted living facilities mandated the two-dose herpes zoster vaccine for all residents (all were well over 50 years of age). Vaccinations were rolled out according to alphabetical order of each resident's last name. After about half the residents were vaccinated, the mandate was successfully challenged by the daughter of one of the residents, and mandatory vaccination was stopped (voluntary vaccination continued, of course). Many of the residents are still alive today, and many have passed on. Some were dementia-free in 2013. Others had Alzheimer disease or other form of dementia.

Assemble an outline for an approach section, assuming your aims are (1) to identify surviving patients who had received or didn't receive the vaccine in 2013 and (2) to determine if the rate of dementia is lower among those who received the vaccine. Don't worry about supplying a lot of detail, nor about charts, figures, and tables.

Suggested Response

Let's assume the main heading for the approach section is lettered "C."

For C.1, the overall strategy, you can start with an overview. Summarize your methods, including how you will identify the two different groups of patients. (e.g., contacting the facilities, obtaining medical records). You don't need to supply these details for the exercise. Just know the general information that goes under this subheading.

We can continue with any preliminary studies (C.2). Let's assume you haven't carried any out. Prior work by other researchers belongs in the significance section.

Now, you can describe research procedures for your specific aim #1:

C.3 *Identify patients across an assisted living network who had and hadn't received herpes zoster vaccine in 2013 during a temporarily mandated vaccine campaign, and who were dementia-free.*

Now you can proceed with subheadings under this aim. Each should describe an important procedure or something about the research participants or setting. You can make up any details you wish for this exercise or simply create a basic outline such as this one:

C.3.1 Description of the assisted living network
C.3.2 Description of the vaccine campaign and rollout and the natural experiment it created
C.3.3 Description of the vaccine (e.g., manufacturer, dosage)
C.3.4 Review of medical records to ensure patients were dementia-free during 2013 (the year the campaign was stopped)

Now it's time to consider the second aim:

C.4 *Measure the rate of dementia of all types among patients who were and were not vaccinated in the network in 2013.*

    C.4.1   Confirmation of diagnosis: You may wish to describe how a diagnosis of dementia (the sole outcome of the study) was determined, and just as importantly the timeframe over which the diagnosis was recorded. For example, a patient may have been vaccinated in 2013 and diagnosed with dementia a week later. It's unlikely the vaccine had anything to do with the diagnosis. So a timeframe of, say, 2018 to 2025 might be appropriate. Diagnoses may be extracted from medical records.

We can complete our outline with sections similar to those in Rahul's scenario.

C.5 *Sample size, power, and statistical analyses*: In this section you would provide support that you have an adequate number of research participants to demonstrate a meaningful difference in dementia rates. A description of how the data you collect will be statistically analyzed should be included. You can use separate subheadings if you wish for sample size, power, and statistical analyses.

C.6 *Challenges and alternative strategies*: In this section, you could address anticipated problems such as research participants who have moved away, have incomplete medical records, didn't receive both doses of the vaccine, etc. It's important to acknowledge these problems even if you don't have effective solutions. For example, patients with incomplete records could just be excluded from the analyses, just like patients who received only one dose of vaccine.

12

Writing for Non-Experts

You may wonder why I've included a chapter on writing for "non-experts." After all, this book is about scientific writing, and scientific writing is meant to be read by those with at least some expertise and interest in the subject matter. There are compelling reasons, however, for learning to write well for non-experts.

Before we discuss the rationale for this chapter, I've chosen the term "non-expert" versus other terms you've certainly heard of, including "lay audience," "non-scientific "audience, or "general public." "Lay" comes from Middle English and originally meant uneducated or not belonging to the clergy. "Non-scientific" isn't really accurate for the content of this chapter. At times, the type of people who read your scientific writing might be scientists themselves but don't have any significant background in the specific content. It wouldn't be fair to called them "non-scientific," though they may be "non-experts." "General public" is a greatly overused term, one that I've always thought of as meaningless. The public is diverse in its education, knowledge, interests, and ability to understand complex information. There really is no "general public." Instead, as we'll discuss, when writing for non-experts, you should carefully consider the specific audience you are targeting. "Non-experts" are simply those with little or no knowledge of the field in which you have a great deal of knowledge.

Here are some important reasons to develop and apply skills in writing for non-experts:

1. On many occasions you will need to write for non-experts to help them understand your work. Imagine that a journalist has reached out to you about some interesting findings and asks for a quick email summary of your research and why it's important for patients. You can't just cut and paste the abstract from your recent research paper—the reporter probably won't understand it, nor will her readers. Imagine also that you have assembled a community advisory board that provides guidance about how to recruit patients for your research, and you need to send them quarterly summaries of your research progress. These summaries need

to be written in a way that non-experts can understand. There are many other examples where you might need to write for non-experts, such as preparing patient education materials, research consent forms, etc.

2. You will often be *required* to write for non-experts. Granting bodies in the United States and the United Kingdom, for example, require plain language or plain English summaries of research. Many agencies within the U.S. government are required to provide instructions and other materials in plain language, which is defined as clear language that the public can easily understand and use.[1]

3. Writing for non-experts helps others gauge the quality and impact of your work. For example, though many grant application review panelists have considerable expertise in the applications they review, a plain language summary that emphasizes the most salient points will help them to assess the importance of your work. In other words, writing a compelling plain language summary makes for a stronger proposal. As a reviewer from the National Institute for Health and Care Research in the United Kingdom commented, "If the plain English summary is well-written, somehow the whole application seems easier to assess—I have an idea of what it is about."[2]

4. A final reason the skills in this chapter are important is well aligned with the rest of the content of this book. The 5Cs are highly applicable to writing for non-experts. Simple, plain language is easy to understand for everyone, and you should use as much of it as often as you can, whether writing for non-experts or not. I also believe the ability to explain things in plain language is useful for clarifying your own ideas. You can't throw in too much jargon into plain language materials. Instead, you have to determine how to explain the jargon in the simplest terms, which may help you yourself clarify its meaning.

If you are a health care professional, you almost certainly already have the ability to communicate with an important group of non-experts: patients. Nearly every day I do my best to communicate health-related information to my patients in a way that they can understand and that helps to engage them in their own care. A couple of weeks before writing this chapter, an elderly man came to see me experiencing episodic shortness of breath and rapid heartbeat.

---

[1] National Institutes of Health. https://www.nih.gov/institutes-nih/nih-office-director/office-communications-public-liaison/clear-communication/plain-language/plain-language-getting-started-or-brushing. Accessed August 14, 2024.

[2] National Institute of Health Research. https://www.learningforinvolvement.org.uk/wp-content/uploads/2021/04/Plain-English-Summaries-2022.pdf. Accessed August 14, 2024.

The result of a 3-day heart monitor test revealed "More than 50 episodes of paroxysmal SVT, most likely due to atrioventricular nodal re-entrant tachycardia." He was able to view this result in his electronic health record and had the natural questions: What does this mean? Is it serious? What can be done about it?

My explanation, carefully practiced over many years of communicating similar information, included, "You have times when your heart beats very rapidly for a few seconds. This might be because there is an electric circuit within your heart that is causing it to fire more often than it needs to." Some of you might have done better, but my explanation of his diagnosis was satisfactory to him, and he also felt reassured that his condition could be managed and wasn't life-threatening. My point is that many of us communicate complex information to non-experts daily, and those of us who write should be able to do so in our writing as well.

Let's say you're not a clinician and you have no contact with patients, but you carry out research in a laboratory. If your child, or mother, or someone else you're close to asks you to explain your research, you will almost certainly avoid complicated jargon and make no assumptions about what they already understand. Though we do our best to communicate complex information in plain language verbally, for some reason, when many people try to put things down on paper, we struggle to communicate plainly, and our explanations can become incomprehensible to non-experts. I believe this is because we get so caught up and excited by our own work, and we mostly communicate about it to people in the field. When we write for non-experts, we sometimes forget that our audience cannot understand things that we consider to be very basic.

Fortunately, there is a large amount of advice available from many sources to guide us in writing for non-experts. Advice is generally consistent among experts in scientific communication, organizations, and countries. I've distilled the advice into a finite set of common principles. Let's assume that what you'll need to write for non-experts is a summary of proposed or completed research. Many of the principles are applicable to other types of writing, such as patient education materials, consent forms, etc.

1. *Identify your audience.* As I noted above, there is no such thing as the "general public." How you write for a group of government policymakers will be quite different than how you write for a patient with low health literacy. The first step, if not already well defined, is to make note of who exactly your writing piece is intended for.
2. *Start with the bottom line or conclusions.* When you write a scientific abstract or a specific aims section, as we've discussed, you generally start with some background and rationale for the research. But when

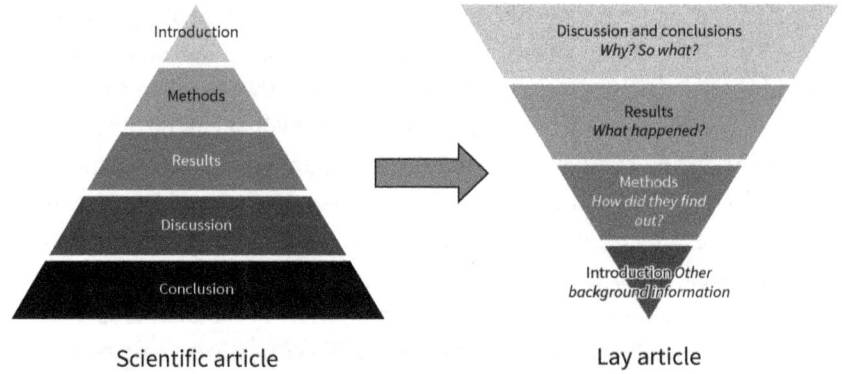

Figure 12.1 Contrast between communications intended for a scientific versus a non-expert (lay) audience. Salita describes the two styles as a pyramid and inverted pyramid.

writing for non-experts, as Kristin Sainani of Stanford recommends, "Start with the take-home message."[3] She offers the example of an abstract for a research paper on generating fresh liquid water from the atmosphere. The scientific abstract begins, "Atmospheric water is a resource equivalent to approximately 10% of all fresh water in lakes on Earth." The non-expert version begins, "Scientists have created a device that can pull water out of air." It is easier to capture a non-expert's attention with the "bottom line" rather than beginning with a rationale and background, even if that's the order in which we are accustomed to receiving information. Joselita Salita goes further and contrasts a scientific article with a "lay" or non-expert article as a pyramid and an inverted pyramid (Figure 12.1).[4]

3. *Avoid jargon whenever possible.* This seemingly obvious advice is easy to overlook when we are immersed in the complexities of scientific writing. When jargon is unavoidable, define it precisely and simply. Avoid using abbreviations and acronyms, even if they are very familiar to others in your field. This principle is, of course, aligned with the 5Cs principle of "commonness." In many cases, commonly used medical terms have equivalents that are better understand by non-experts, such as "high blood pressure" for hypertension and "heart attack" for myocardial infarction. Keep in mind, however, that some terms commonly used in biomedical literature have a different meaning for non-experts; in such

[3] ACS Webinars. https://www.acs.org/acs-webinars/library/write-well-and-prosper-science-writing-tips-sainani.html. Accessed August 14, 2024.
[4] Salita, J. Writing for lay audiences: A challenge for scientists. Med Writing 2015;24(4):183–189.

Table 12.1 Scientific Terms and Equivalents for Non-Experts

Scientific Term	Meaning for Lay Audiences	Suggested Equivalent for Lay Audiences
Significant	Important	Did not happen by chance
Fraction	Small part	A part
Trauma	Psychological event	Physical damage
Enhance	Improve	Intensify, increase
Positive trend	Good trend	Upward trend
Positive feedback	Good response, praise	Vicious cycle, self-reinforcing
Theory	Hunch, speculation	Scientific understanding
Uncertainty	Ignorance	Range
Error	Mistake, wrong, incorrect	Difference from true value
Values	Ethics, monetary value	Numbers, quantity
Scheme	Devious plot	Systematic plan
Anomaly	Abnormal occurrence	Change from long-term average

cases, alternative terms are preferred. Salita provides an excellent table with such commonly used terms and alternatives (Table 12.1).[4]

4. *Use positive words and statements.* Positive words and statements are easier to understand, and this recommendation is, of course, aligned with the principle of cogency. The National Institutes of Health (NIH) offers the following very simple example:[5] "Don't forget to refill your prescription" is not as cogent as "Remember to refill you prescription."

5. *Keep sentences short and include only necessary information.* In other words, follow the principle of conciseness. The NIH recommends no more than 20 words per sentence.[6] Your audience may get lost with longer sentences. There is also a strong temptation to include all the details you would include in a scientific piece in a piece for non-experts. Some details are simply not needed for non-experts. Use your discretion about including them.

6. *Avoid padding.* Aligned with the principle of cogency, "padding" refers to words such as "very," "really," "actually, etc. that don't really serve any purpose and can zap the power out of a sentence. The NIH offers the

---

[5] National Institutes of Health. https://www.nih.gov/institutes-nih/nih-office-director/office-communications-public-liaison/clear-communication/plain-language/plain-language-getting-started-or-brushing. Accessed August 10, 2024.

[6] National Institutes of Health. https://www.nih.gov/institutes-nih/nih-office-director/office-communications-public-liaison/clear-communication/plain-language/plain-language-getting-started-or-brushing. Accessed August 10, 2024.

example of "rare but potentially very deadly conditions at birth," which could be rewritten as "rare but potentially deadly conditions."[7] "Very" is unnecessary.

7. *Use the active voice.* Again, align with the principle of cogency. The active voice is especially important in making an impact on a non-expert audience—for example, "We found treatment B to be better at preventing stroke" versus "Treatment B was found to be better at preventing stroke."

8. *Organize your text for maximum clarity.* Aligned with the principles of both clarity and consistency, use bulleted lists, bolded headings, and short paragraphs. These tools make your message easier to understand.

9. *Use a readability test.* Readability tests identify how difficult a passage is to read and the level of education required to understand it. Many of these tests are based on Flesch's and Kincaid's readability formula.[8] You can check the Flesch–Kincaid Grade Level of your work in the "Spelling and Grammar" review feature within Microsoft Word (see also below). Alternatively, there are several places online where you can check the readability of your text, such as http://read-able.com. Revise your piece if needed and check it again until it's readable for your target audience.

10. *Ask members of your target audience to read your piece.* This is a critical final step in preparing your piece for non-experts. Ask at least one non-expert to read it. You will be surprised how often things that seem obvious to you will be unclear to a non-expert. Revise accordingly.

I would encourage you also to use visual aids (also called "visuals"), such as simple figures, tables, and pictures, to help your audience understand your message. Include them generously. There is a whole science of how to communicate health information by using visuals, which can help emphasize the message you write about or even replace parts of it. The Centers for Disease Control and Prevention (CDC) has an excellent inventory of resources.[9] But this book and this chapter are about writing, not designing visuals, so I haven't devoted too much space to visuals.

---

[7] National Institutes of Health. https://www.nih.gov/institutes-nih/nih-office-director/office-communi cations-public-liaison/clear-communication/plain-language/plain-language-getting-started-or-brushing. Accessed August 10, 2024.

[8] Kincaid JP, Fishburne RP, Rogers RL, Chissom BS. *Derivation of new readability formulas (automated readability index, fog count, and Flesch reading ease formula) for Navy enlisted personnel.* Research Branch Report 8–75. Chief of Naval Technical Training: Naval Air Station Memphis, 1975.

[9] Centers for Disease Control and Prevention. https://www.cdc.gov/healthliteracy/developmaterials/vis ual-communication.html. Accessed August 14, 2023.

Scenario: *Ivan and his colleagues have developed a new malaria vaccine (Prev-Mal R19) and evaluated its safety and efficacy among children at risk for malaria living in Cameroon, Africa. The advantage of Prev-Mal R19 is that it is stable at temperatures under 35 degrees Celsius and doesn't require continuous refrigeration, unlike other available vaccines. It is administered in three doses to children at age 12 months, 18 months, and 2 years. Ivan and his team have published their work in a prominent infectious diseases journal. Ivan is seeking support to expand this promising work and needs to write an abstract that can be easily understood by potential donors to the foundation that supports the research. The abstract can be no more than 100 words long.*

Here is Ivan's scientific abstract:

Background: *Malaria is a significant global challenge. Children in endemic areas of sub-Saharan Africa are especially vulnerable. Two vaccines have been approved by the WHO to prevent malaria infection. Unfortunately, though effective, both require storage between 2 and 8 degrees Celsius, which presents a significant logistical and resource challenge in regions where the vaccines are most needed. Prev-Mal R19 is a new malaria vaccine that doesn't require refrigeration. This study is an evaluation of the efficacy and safety of Prev-Mal R19 in a randomized-controlled trial.*

Methods: *The trial was conducted across five distinct regions of Cameroon with different baseline incidence of malaria and differing seasonal variation in infection. Children age less than 1 year of age were randomly assigned (ratio 2:1) to Prev-Mal R19 10 ug administered at age 12 months, 18 months, and 2 years or control vaccine (rabies vaccine). Families, vaccine administrators, and local research personnel were all masked to treatment allocation. The primary outcome was incidence of malaria. Secondary outcomes included hospitalizations for and deaths from malaria and vaccine side effects. All outcomes were measured over 36 months following administration of the final dose in the series.*

Results: *Between August 2021 and September 2024, 6,320 children were enrolled in the study. 4,235 were allocated to the Prev-Mal R19 arm. A total of 3,610 children received all doses in the series for both vaccines (2,390 in the Prev-Mal R19 arm and 1,220 in the control arm). Side effects were minimal in both groups, with injection site irritation and fever being most common. The incidence of side effects did not differ significantly between the two groups. Vaccine efficacy over 36 months for Prev-Mal R19 was 80% (95% CI, 76%, 84%).*

Among those infected by malaria, Prev-Mal R19 was associated with a reduction in risk for hospitalization of 60% (95% CI, 42%, 78%). There were no vaccine- or malaria-related deaths in the study.

Conclusion: *Prev-Mal R19 is highly effective and safe for prevention of malaria in children. It is useful as a more practical alternative to other malaria vaccines.*

Ivan follows a systematic approach to writing his very short (100 words) abstract. First, his audience consists of potential donors and foundation officers. These are likely to be well-educated people with some knowledge of health matters, if not vaccines and malaria. This allows Ivan to use more complex language than in an abstract intended for a less educated audience. Nevertheless, there is nothing wrong with keeping things as simple as possible.

He should start with the bottom-line message, such as:

Prev-Mal R19 is a new, effective, and safe vaccine against the serious problem of malaria in children.

Notice that this opening sentence not only incorporates the bottom line but also provides a bit of background by emphasizing the seriousness of malaria in children. He could then continue with a short sentence on the rationale for the study:

Two effective vaccines are already approved against malaria, but, unlike Prev-Mal R19, both require refrigeration.

He could continue with a short sentence on what he and his team accomplished. Notice the active voice:

We determined the effectiveness and safety of Prev-Mal R19 by comparing it to a vaccine for rabies that has no effect in preventing malaria.

There is lots of information in the methods and results sections that isn't needed for Ivan's audience, such as the dosage schedule, the randomization ratio, etc. Including a few numbers, such as the number of children enrolled and the period of follow-up, is reasonable:

We enrolled 6,320 children and followed them for 36 months.

The vaccine effectiveness is simply the reduction in risk of infection with the vaccine under study. This can be phrased as:

Prev-Mal R19 reduced the risk of malaria infection by 80%.

There is no need to give the confidence intervals, which the audience would probably not understand.

Ivan could include a couple of sentences on secondary outcomes:

Among children who did get malaria, those who got Prev-Mal R19 had a 60% lower risk of being admitted to the hospital. No children died, and side effects were mild.

Since he started with the conclusion/bottom line, there is no need to include anything more. Here is his complete abstract:

Prev-Mal R19 is a new, effective, and safe vaccine against the serious problem of malaria in children. Two effective vaccines are already approved against malaria, but, unlike Prev-Mal R19, both require refrigeration. We determined the effectiveness and safety of Prev-Mal R19 by comparing it to a vaccine for rabies that has no effect in preventing malaria. We enrolled 6,320 children and followed them for 36 months. Prev-Mal R19 reduced the risk of malaria infection by 80%. Among children who did get malaria, those who got Prev-Mal R19 had a 60% lower risk of being admitted to the hospital. No children died, and side effects were mild. (98 words)

A friend from outside the health care field whom Ivan asked to read over his summary found it to be easily understood. The Flesch–Kincaid reading grade level is 10.7, according to the tool available in the "Spelling and Grammar" toolkit in Microsoft Word (see more on this tool below). Ivan believes this is acceptable for his audience.

Table 12.2 provides a short summary of the application of the 5Cs to writing for non-experts.

Writing for Non-Experts Exercise

The following scientific abstract is from an article entitled "Safety and Immunogenicity of a Single-Shot Live-Attenuated Chikungunya Vaccine: A Double-Blind, Multicentre, Randomised, Placebo-Controlled, Phase 3 Trial,"

Table 12.2 5Cs and Writing for Non-Experts

Conciseness	Short sentences are easier to understand. Keep sentence to less than 20 words whenever possible. Don't include details that aren't necessary for non-experts.
Cogency	As always, use the active voice and put statements in positive form—for instance, "We recruited 100 people" instead of "100 people were recruited" and "Remember to exercise daily" instead of "Don't forget to exercise daily."
Clarity	Good ways to achieve clarity include getting someone from your target audience to read over your work and to make edits if anything is unclear. Visuals can help with clarity.
Commonness	Avoid acronyms and unfamiliar abbreviations. Always check the readability level of your piece.
Consistency	Start with the bottom-line message. Use headings (included bolded headings) and bullets generously. Organize your piece into short paragraphs or passages. This makes it easier for your audience to follow and is consistent with how a wide variety of information is presented. (e.g., safety information on an airplane). Use visuals if possible.

which was published in the prestigious journal *Lancet* in 2023.[10] Your task is to use the information to write a 100-word unstructured abstract intended for those who might read about the study on a general news website. Your non-expert abstract should be easily understood by those with a high school education or less. You may wish to include a short sentence on the disease chikungunya (a quick internet search will reveal lots of useful information).

Background: *VLA1553 is a live-attenuated vaccine candidate for active immunisation and prevention of disease caused by chikungunya virus. We report safety and immunogenicity data up to day 180 after vaccination with VLA1553.*

Methods: *This double-blind, multicentre, randomised, phase 3 trial was done in 43 professional vaccine trial sites in the USA. Eligible participants were healthy volunteers aged 18 years and older. Patients were excluded if they had history of chikungunya virus infection or immune-mediated or chronic arthritis or arthralgia, known or suspected defect of the immune system, any inactivated vaccine received within 2 weeks before vaccination with VLA1553, or any live vaccine received within 4 weeks before vaccination with VLA1553. Participants were randomised (3:1) to receive VLA1553 or placebo. The primary endpoint was the proportion of baseline negative participants with a seroprotective chikungunya virus antibody level defined as 50% plaque reduction in a micro*

[10] Schneider M, Narciso-Abraham M, Hadl S, et al. Safety and immunogenicity of a single-shot live-attenuated chikungunya vaccine: A double-blind, multicentre, randomised, placebo-controlled, phase 3 trial. Lancet 2023Jun 24;401(10394):2138–2147. doi:10.1016/S0140-6736(23)00641-4. Epub 2023 Jun 12. PMID: 37321235; PMCID: OMC13014240.

plaque reduction neutralisation test (μPRNT) with a μPRNT$_{50}$ titre of at least 150, 28 days after vaccination. The safety analysis included all individuals who received vaccination. Immunogenicity analyses were done in a subset of participants at 12 pre-selected study sites. These participants were required to have no major protocol deviations to be included in the per-protocol popula-tion for immunogenicity analyses. This trial is registered at ClinicalTrials.gov, NCT04546724.

Findings: Between Sept 17, 2020 and April 10, 2021, 6100 people were screened for eligibility. 1972 people were excluded and 4128 participants were enrolled and randomised (3093 to VLA1553 and 1035 to placebo). 358 participants in the VLA1553 group and 133 participants in the placebo group discontinued be-fore trial end. The per-protocol population for immunogenicity analysis com-prised 362 participants (266 in the VLA1553 group and 96 in the placebo group). After a single vaccination, VLA1553 induced seroprotective chikungunya virus neutralising antibody levels in 263 (98·9%) of 266 participants in the VLA1553 group (95% CI 96·7-99·8; p<0·0001) 28 days post-vaccination, independent of age. VLA1553 was generally safe with an adverse event profile similar to other licensed vaccines and equally well tolerated in younger and older adults. Serious adverse events were reported in 46 (1·5%) of 3082 participants exposed to VLA1553 and eight (0·8%) of 1033 participants in the placebo arm. Only two serious adverse events were considered related to VLA1553 treatment (one mild myalgia and one syndrome of inappropriate antidiuretic hormone secre-tion). Both participants recovered fully.

Interpretation: The strong immune response and the generation of seroprotective titres in almost all vaccinated participants suggests that VLA1553 is an excellent candidate for the prevention of disease caused by chi-kungunya virus.

Suggested Response

You have just 100 words, and there is a great deal of information that the target audience may neither wish to nor need to know. As noted above, it's probably best to include a short sentence describing chikungunya. Here is a possible paragraph:

VLA1553, a new vaccine for chikungunya, produces a good immune response and is safe. Chikungunya is a viral infection, most common in Africa and Asia, that is spread by mosquitoes and causes headache, joint and muscle pain, and rash. We compared VLA1553 to a placebo vaccine. We enrolled 4,128 people and analyzed the immune response in 362 of them (266 in the vaccine group and 96 in the placebo group). 98.9% of people in the vaccine group developed protective antibodies across all age groups. Only 2 people developed serious vaccine side effects. Our results support VLA1553 for chikungunya prevention. (98 words)

Notice that the suggested response begins with the bottom line. Alternatively, you could begin with a description of chikungunya, since most people are not familiar with it, and then include the bottom line. Certain details such as "live-attenuated virus" are unnecessary for non-experts. As a test, you can ask a non-expert to read the paragraph and then ask them to report their understanding. If it's accurate and reasonably complete, you've done a good job. To assess readability, highlight your paragraph in Microsoft Word and click on Review → Spelling and Grammar on the top menu ribbon. Click on "Spelling and Grammar" once again. This should bring up the "Editor," which provides a score, etc. Since the piece is intended for non-experts, select "casual writing" to identify any spelling and grammar suggestions. You will find the Flesch–Kincaid readability grade level under Insights → Document stats. In this case the grade level is in the range of a ninth-grade level, appropriate for the target audience.

13

Developing a Writing Habit

I hope you've found the recommendations in this book useful so far. There is, of course, no point in studying them, reflecting about them, or committing them to memory without applying them to actual writing. In other words, this book isn't about theory, but practical application, which is why I've included the exercises. Practical application means regular practice—writing often. For anyone in the biomedical fields, finding something to write shouldn't be a problem. In fact, the number of opportunities to write for any individual often exceeds one's ability to take advantage of them. That ability is constrained not just by a lack of skill and knowledge, which we've covered extensively, and of which I provided a detailed example in the introduction, but by one's ability to forge a regular writing habit. The *Oxford English Dictionary* defines a habit as a constant, almost automatic, practice acquired by frequent repetition.[1] For most people, however, acquiring writing as a "constant, almost automatic practice" is a long way off.

There is no shortage of advice available on developing a writing habit, including how and when to write, where to write, how much to write, and even what to write about while developing a habit. Much of this advice is simply one man's or one woman's opinion. As you can imagine, how to develop a writing habit isn't subject to the same rigorous, scientific approach as the content of what you write about. Like the many books, websites, and other resources available about writing habits, I could also add my "two cents" about what I believe works. And, of course, like others who have written about the topic, it would inevitably be what works for *me*. Fortunately, however, there is a small body of work that constitutes the science of how to develop a writing habit. In this chapter, where there are gaps in the science, I do offer my opinion, based on my many years of teaching scientific writing. Ultimately, what I recommend may or may not work for you, but I urge you to at least give it a try.

Much of what we know about being a productive writer of any kind is based on the work of Robert Boice, a professor of psychology and education who has studied writing productivity for decades and who carried out an influential

---

[1] https://www.oed.com/?tl=true

experiment in the 1980s. Boice began with the hypothesis that being a productive writer indeed involves making writing a regular, daily habit that one essentially forces oneself to carry out.[2] He questioned the value of waiting for inspiration to stimulate the desire to write, believing that waiting for the mood to strike would lead to little output. There was already some support for his ideas. Boice points out the work of John D. Gould of IBM's research division, who noted that professional writers have a longstanding daily preoccupation with writing.[3] Boice also found support in the work of Jerome Bruner, who believed that writing is an experience that nourishes itself and, through practice, helps develop problem-solving mechanisms.[4]

With his well-developed convictions and this support, Boice carried out "An Experiment on 'Produced Writing and Creativity.'" He recruited 27 academicians from local colleges in southern California who expressed a desire to be more productive writers and agreed to participate in the 10-week study. At baseline, the participants described their writing productivity and then agreed to establish a regular writing schedule 5 days a week, to log how much they wrote, and to record the creative ideas they had for writing. Most subjects reported fewer than four creative ideas per day. It's not clear to me exactly what constituted a creative idea. Four certainly sounds like a significant number to me; I'd be pleased if I could come up with one or two. Boice offers the inscrutable example of "a new realization that two previously developed ideas for writing could be connected" as a creative idea.

Nine of the participants were placed in what he called the control group, who agreed to defer any writing for 10 weeks. In most biomedical study designs, of course, a control group would be more like a "usual care" situation: Participants would be asked to continue to write in their usual way, while still logging their progress, rather than consciously avoiding writing. Another nine participants were assigned to a group Boice called "spontaneous writing." They were told to write according to a schedule when they felt like it for 3 weeks. In other words, they were expected to write according to the schedule if the mood struck them, and not to write otherwise. Beginning in Week 4, the members of this group were told to write more at each scheduled time in which they chose to write at all.

The third group of nine was assigned to a *contingency* condition. They were asked to write a minimum of three pages daily. If that output was not achieved

[2] Boice R. The neglected third factor in writing productivity. College Composition and Communication 1985;36(4):472–480.
[3] Gould JD. Experiments in composing letters. In: Gregg L, Steinberg E (eds.), *Cognitive processes in writing*. Lawrence Erlbaum, 1980.
[4] Bruner J. *On knowing: Essays for the left hand*. Belknap Press of Harvard University Press, 1979.

Table 13.1 Writing Output: Mean Number of Pages per Scheduled/Potential Working Day

Group	Before Scheduled Writing Phase	Scheduled Writing Phase
Control	0.1	0.2
Spontaneous	0.3	0.9
Contingency	0.4	3.2

on a daily basis, they had to write a check to a despised organization for $15. The example Boice provides in his paper was the Ku Klux Klan.

I find the conditions in Boice's experiment problematic for a couple of reasons. First, if the possibility of having to write a check to the KKK was part of the experiment, I wouldn't participate, and I'm guessing many others wouldn't either. Second, $15 a day for college academicians in the 1980s is an awfully severe punishment even without the requirement to send the money to a despised organization. Boice would have been better off taking advantage of the behavioral economic principle of "loss aversion."[5] The nine contingency participants could each have started with a $100 stipend for participation, and to return a certain amount, say $5, on days when they didn't meet the output goal.

I won't leave you in suspense too long. Boice summarized his results in Table 13.1. The number of creative ideas showed a similar gradient among the three groups. I don't think the results are surprising, though I *am* a little surprised that participants told not to write still managed 0.2 pages per day!

Boice concludes that the greatest levels of both writing productivity and creativity came under the condition where writing was forced. He also states that "good writing depends on frequent practice, independent of the writer's mood" and that "where students become habitual writers, a surprising amount of learning to write may take of itself."

Boice's impressive results are largely the foundation for the longstanding recommendation that being a productive writer requires making writing a daily habit, to which one must be as committed as any other professional activity. Indeed, Boice's work plays an important role in Paul Silvia's book, *How to Write a Lot: A Practical Guide to Productive Academic Writing*, published by

---

[5] Rao G, Krall J, Loewenstein G. An internet-based pediatric weight management program with and without financial incentives: A randomized trial. Child Obes 2011;7(2):122–128.

the American Psychological Association.[6] While, as I'll discuss later, I believe writing daily is a good way for novice biomedical writers to be productive, and one I adopted long ago, as I've indicated, I find Boice's experiment problematic as a source of evidence for this recommendation. Punishing the contingency participants for not meeting an output target is not a realistic situation, and I wonder, as you might as well, about the quality of the work they produced.

Helen Sword of the University of Auckland, New Zealand, published an important article in 2016 entitled " 'Write Every Day!': A Mantra Dismantled."[7] In it she states, "Remove Boice from the equation, and the existing literature on scholarly writing offers little or no conclusive evidence that academics who write every day are any more prolific, productive, or otherwise successful than those who do not."

Sword questions the validity of the methods and conclusions of Boice's experiment, in the same way that I have in this chapter to a lesser extent. Her more important contribution, however, is her analysis of 100 interviews she carried out among successful academic writers. Among the 100, "only two described writing routines that closely resemble Boice's recommended regime of scheduling daily sequestered writing time." Sword found that successful academic writers have a variety of different styles of committing time to writing, including "binge writing," the practice of writing intensely over short periods, a practice Boice and others explicitly discourage. Sword concludes,

> The bottom line is that Boice's austere methods do not reflect—and in some cases are antithetical to—the real-life practice of productive academics. For the vast majority of colleagues I interviewed, writing is neither a daily routine nor a rare occurrence, neither an immovable constant nor a random event, neither a public activity nor a rigidly sequestered one; writing is the work that gets done in the interstices between teaching, office hours, faculty meetings, administration, email, family events, and all the other messy sprawling demands of academic life.

So what is one to make of Boice's experiment and advice and Sword's contradictory findings? I think the two perspectives can be reconciled by distinguishing between those who are already prolific writers and those who are starting out or otherwise struggle for whatever reason. For example, as an example of a binge writer, Sword quotes Steven Pinker, a hugely productive professor of psychology at Harvard, and hardly a novice. Though I write daily,

---

[6] Silvia PT. *How to write a lot: A practical guide to productive academic writing*. American Psychological Association, APA LifeTools, 2019.
[7] Sword H. "Write every day!": A mantra dismantled. International Journal of Academic Development 2016;21(4):312–322.

I have also adopted many of the habits Sword describes, as I write between meetings and patient encounters, and sometimes in loud, crowded places. In fact, I wrote the first part of this chapter at Ronald Reagan National Airport in Washington, DC as I waited for a flight.

While Sword is critical of Boice's work and has found a diversity of writing habits among successful writers, she herself states, "These days, I still write nearly every weekday before breakfast." She also writes that many of the strategies recommended by Boice, Silvia, and others have worked for her. I also write nearly every day, early in the morning, and when that isn't possible, I find anywhere from 30 minutes to an hour during the rest of the day to write. So while Sword has sort of dismantled the "write every day" mantra, I have little doubt that a disciplined daily writing habit is the best way for you, unless you are already prolific, to be productive.

While Boice and Sword provide somewhat of an analytical or scientific approach to the keys to productivity about how often and when to write, advice about other aspects of writing is largely based on the opinions of a few who have thought carefully about them. I've added my thoughts to this chorus to come up with the following recommendations:

1. *How often to write*: As I've noted above, I write daily, as do other productive writers. Daily writing according to a strict schedule is an essential part of advice from Boice and Silvia. I would advise that daily writing isn't necessary, but that writing according to a regular schedule is an important driver of productivity. Sometimes writing daily just isn't possible for many people in biomedical fields. If you are one of them, try scheduling two or three writing sessions per week.

2. *When to write*: I prefer early mornings, simply because writing is an activity that requires intense concentration and a well-rested mind. It works for me, and if you're not yet sure what works for you, I advise you to try it. The trouble with trying to write later in the day, between meetings and clinical care or after a long tough day, is that there are simply too many distractions that suck up both time and energy. It becomes easier to blame other activities for the failure to be productive. Instead, aim to write as early as possible—for me, that's between 6 and 7 a.m., 7 days a week.

3. *Where to write*: Write in a very quiet, well-lit place—although some dispute what sounds like obvious advice. Writing is and should be a solitary activity. I know many laptops are open in coffee shops and other places, and I've already confessed to writing in a busy airport (mainly because I had nothing else to do), but I assure you that writing in a quiet place

with no other distractions is best. Multitasking is popular, especially among younger generations, but there is no shortage of evidence that it simply doesn't work.[8] You can't listen to music and write at the same time. You can't people watch at a coffee shop every few minutes while writing. And you can't monitor your social media feeds and respond regularly while writing. Find a quiet room with no one around. Nothing but a word processing program should be open on your computer (antivirus software and other background applications are exceptions, of course). If you're accustomed to multitasking or a noisier environment while trying to write, you'll be surprised at how much more productive you are in a quiet room.

4. *How much to write*: There is no simple answer to this. Boice's research participants were forced to be productive, but, as I've stated, I worry about the quality of work when one is forced to meet some target. I also don't believe in a time-based target of, say, 30 minutes or 1 hour. As you write, I think you'll reach a point where you believe you've done a decent amount of writing for a session. For less experienced biomedical writers, I think about 300 to 400 words in a session is reasonable (which could be completed in 1 hour or less). It may be less than that if you're inserting many citations, which is time-consuming (citations shouldn't count toward your word total), or trying to explain technical jargon as carefully as possible. I think it's more important to write *something* during each session rather than trying to meet a strict page or word count or time limit.

5. *What to write about*: The answer to this question is complicated.
   a. There's no doubt than any academic in the biomedical fields will, at least from time to time, be obliged to write papers, abstracts, etc. based on the results of original research or for some other reason.
   b. There are also those of you who don't have these obligations right now but, I hope, have become enthusiastic about writing after reading this book. In such cases, you can seek out writing opportunities. There are lots of them, of course, including opportunities to contribute chapters to books, to write review articles, or even just to assist with part of a paper.
   c. The third category of what to write involves even more ambition. Some of you might decide that you want to produce something that is personally meaningful and important, without an obvious place to have it published. Let's say you're passionate about improving dementia

---

[8] Madore KP, Wagner AD. Multicosts of multitasking. Cerebrum 2019 Apr 1;2019:cer-04-19. PMID: 32206165; PMCID: PMC7075496.

care for the elderly and have decided to write a detailed narrative review article about best practices, based on your own experience and a review of the literature. Once you've finished, you could consider submitting it to a journal that accepts unsolicited review articles. It may be turned down and you can try elsewhere. In the worst-case scenario, you can't get it published, but you will still have a body of work you can be proud of and share with colleagues, students, and others.

No matter which of these three categories you fall into, I strongly recommend the following: Focus on one writing project at a time until it's finished! Like multitasking, which doesn't work, I believe that jumping from one project to another, writing a couple of hundred words here or there, is very difficult, as you need to get refocused on each project after being distracted by another.

Now, rather than providing you with an exercise for this chapter, which wouldn't be practical, I offer a case study. It's fictionalized to some extent but is designed to provide you with an idea of how an academic physician could adopt a disciplined and productive approach to scientific writing. I hope it provides some useful strategies as well as a little inspiration.

Case Study

Chua completed her residency training in family medicine in 2019 after having served as chief resident. Having been a "star" resident, she was immediately offered a faculty position in the West River family medicine residency, which has a loose affiliation with a nearby medical school. Her professional activities include direct outpatient and inpatient care, obstetrics, and supervision of family medicine residents, primarily in the outpatient setting. She also leads a weekly case-based conference for the residents. She finds all these activities fulfilling but feels as if a dimension to her career is missing. She is an avid reader of *American Family Physician*, the most widely read journal in the discipline, which provides thorough and timely narrative reviews of topics important to family physicians. The other faculty members in her program have generally not been academically productive, which isn't unusual for community-based programs. Nevertheless, several senior faculty members have encouraged Chua to pursue scientific writing.

She emailed the journal and secured an opportunity to write a narrative review of migraine headache, including epidemiology, diagnosis, and management in primary care settings. Her paper is due 4 months from the time she accepted the opportunity, and, given the tight publishing schedule, there can be no extensions of the deadline. Chua has never written an article before but has read the *Biomedical Writer's Handbook* as well as a couple of other resources on academic writing. She's completed a number of exercises in this book and online. This preparatory work has provided a strong impetus to write, and she is excited about the publication opportunity.

Week 1

Chua identified three times during the week to write: Tuesday, Wednesday, and Friday mornings from 7 to 8 a.m. During her first week, she reached out to a family medicine faculty member in a different program who had previously published an article on headache in *American Family Physician*, as well as a number of other review articles. He agreed to review her paper prior to submission. He left the decision about co-authorship to her, saying, "You can decide if I've been useful enough to be listed." Chua immersed herself in the latest research about migraine, searching for and retrieving 11 articles (3 of which were reviews), and started to think about how to craft an article useful for family physicians. She started to read these articles during her scheduled writing time, highlighting key passages and making careful notes.

Week 2

Chua's background research continued. A bit anxious about the looming deadline, Chua started reading outside of the scheduled writing times. Several of the original 11 articles she retrieved led her to additional articles. By the end of the week, she had read 18 articles, each carefully annotated and highlighted. She placed these in a binder.

Week 3

During her first writing session in Week 3, Chua created a rough outline of her paper:

1. Epidemiology of migraine headache, including prevalence and risk factors

2. Diagnosis of migraine based on accepted criteria; differential diagnosis; challenges to diagnosis in the primary care setting
3. The usefulness of and recommendations for any laboratory testing or radiological imaging
4. Initial management, including lifestyle changes, headache diaries, and pharmacotherapy
5. Additional management considerations for migraine headaches that are refractory to initial management
6. Emerging and future therapies

Chua contemplated her outline for more than half an hour, wondering how to get started. She thought intermittently about her paper between her first and second writing sessions that week.

During her second session, she decided to start writing, knowing that there would be many opportunities for revision. She decided to apply the 5Cs to the best of her ability from the outset, and to avoid immediately revising sections she had written. She began with the opening sentence:

Migraine headache is a common condition that has a profound impact on the quality of life of millions of people.

Not a bad start, Chua thought. She continued with a description of the epidemiology of migraine, writing approximately 300 words by the end of the hour. During her third session that week, she reviewed her notes and papers that described the diagnosis of migraine and began the second section of her paper with:

Migraine is a clinical diagnosis.

She proceeded with briefly describing the International Classification of Headache Disorders diagnostic criteria for migraine in a paragraph. She provided more detail about the criteria in a table. By the end of Week 3, Chua had written a total of 700 words.

Week 4

During her research for her paper, Chua retrieved a number of papers that described the challenges of diagnosis of migraine, including differential diagnosis and the problem of underdiagnosis described in the influential CaMEO-I study.[9] She reread this and several other papers about the challenges of diagnosis, even though she had made careful notes and highlighted passages earlier. She felt that rereading some of the key articles helped her organize a section of the paper on challenges to diagnosis. This second review took up all her writing time during Week 4.

Week 5

Chua set a goal to complete three paragraphs on differential diagnosis and the challenges of diagnosis of migraine in Week 4. She divided this section into three parts: differential diagnosis, underdiagnosis of migraine, and misdiagnosis of migraine. With the relevant background research fresh in her mind, she efficiently wrote a paragraph for each part and completed all three in the first two sessions in Week 5. She used the third writing session to search for any additional relevant papers she may have missed and found none. By the end of Week 5, she had written a total of 1,300 words.

Week 6

As she wrote more and more, Chua became more proficient not only in her writing, but also in organizing relevant information. The greater fluidity made it easy for her to complete a section on laboratory and imaging studies and their indications (usually to rule out other causes of headache). She found a number of key relevant articles that she had already annotated and highlighted. As for the previous section, she reread a couple of these in their entirety and a couple more partially. She was able to complete this section in a session-and-a half. She didn't write at all in her third scheduled session and instead spent some time in the hospital cafeteria with a colleague. Her total word count by the end of Week 6 was 2,100 words.

---

[9] Adams AM, Buse DC, Leroux E, et al. Chronic Migraine Epidemiology and Outcomes—International (CaMEO-I) Study: Methods and multi-country baseline findings for diagnosis rates and care. Cephalalgia 2023;43(6):3331024231180611. doi:10.1177/03331024231180611. PMID: 37314231.

Week 7

During Week 7, Chua was assigned to an inpatient service, where she provided supervision of residents and bedside teaching and also was on call for admissions to the hospital. She kept her writing schedule intact for the week but found herself unable to write, even though she did have time to write before rounding with the residents. She was simply too tired and unable to concentrate sufficiently to write. Also, she had trouble finding a quiet space in the hospital to carry out her work. Furthermore, she felt it best to avoid the anxiety of having to wrap up her writing prior to meeting the residents on time for rounds. Chua did feel a bit guilty about her lack of productivity in Week 7 but resolved to get back to writing in a disciplined, efficient fashion the following week.

Week 8

Eager to sustain her excellent progress, Chua quickly reviewed her notes and papers that described recommendations and guidelines for initial management of migraine headache in her first writing session this week. She began writing in the second session and finished this section in her third session. Her total word count by the end of Week 8 was 2,900 words.

Week 9

With the end of her paper in sight, Chua resolved to come close to finishing in Week 9. She wrote a small section on management of refractory migraines in her first writing session. In sessions two and three, she repeated a search for emerging and future therapies, including searching such resources as ClinicalTrials.gov. She reviewed her notes from the relevant papers she had found initially on emerging and future therapies. Her total word count by the end of the week was 3,200 words.

Week 10

Chua completed her section on emerging and future therapies over the three writing sessions in Week 10. Her total word count was 3,750 words.

Week 11

In her first and second writing sessions of Week 11, Chua wrote a brief, un-structured abstract that met the specifications of *American Family Physician*. In her third session, she read her complete draft and corrected typos and obvious grammatical errors. Most importantly, she looked for any inconsistencies and ambiguities (e.g., unclear diagnostic criteria) and potentially missing information. She made a few small adjustments immediately.

Week 12

Chua applied the 5Cs a second time, making substantial changes especially to improve conciseness and clarity. She completed her revisions by end of the third writing session and had a revised draft version of her paper with a word count of 3,450.

Weeks 13 and 14

Chua shared her draft paper with the senior colleague from another institution. He provided excellent feedback about content, and clarity in particular. He had many suggested changes and edits. He also suggested she include a table on pharmacological options. Grateful for his help, Chua decided to include him as a second author, for which he expressed his thanks. Chua also shared her draft paper with four colleagues from her own program (including two residents), who agreed to read it over and provide feedback within 2 weeks. Only two colleagues actually provided any feedback, the others stating that they unfortunately became too busy to meet Chua's deadline. One of her colleagues, a senior resident, provided detailed comments, including suggestions to improve clarity, which she greatly appreciated. The other colleague, a senior faculty member, also provided detailed comments especially on her section about the challenge of diagnosis of migraine in primary care.

Week 15

Chua incorporated her colleagues' suggestions in a final draft during her first and second writing sessions. During her third session, she submitted her paper to the journal and took a walk at a nearby park while listening to music.

Epilogue

Three months later, Chua received notice from *American Family Physician* that her paper was essentially sound and helpful but would need a few revisions. The editor suggested including a summary section on recommendations for practice as well as a few other relatively minor changes. Enthusiastic about the strong prospect of publication, Chua revised the paper promptly, within 2 weeks. She received an acceptance letter just 2 weeks later.

14
Writing for Wellness

Why do we write in the biomedical professions? The obvious reasons have been made clear directly or indirectly throughout this book—to advance professionally, to disseminate important ideas, to secure funding for new ideas, because it is required for some reason, and to experience the personal satisfaction of publication. All these are compelling reasons, of course, and one or more probably explains why you chose to read this book. Scientific writing is rewarding because of the benefits it brings. Are there other reasons people write? I write daily not only because I often have to, but also because I enjoy it. I not only teach scientific writing but I'm also an editor and a novelist. I also teach creative writing to health care professionals. I teach creative writing because I want others to experience the enjoyment I experience. But there is another important reason some of us write, or some of us *should* write: Writing can be a useful way to cope with the stresses of our professional and personal lives. This is something I discovered first-hand.

You're probably familiar with the widespread phenomenon of burnout among health care professionals, a problem that has received a great deal of attention in recent years. The problem has been studied extensively. Young, old, male, female experienced and inexperienced doctors and nurses all experience burnout at high rates, and the problem has gotten steadily worse. So, like many health care systems, mine decided to address the problem systematically. The first task was to appoint someone to lead the effort. We were not at all unique in this regard: Just about every large health care system, both academic health systems and others, has in recent years appointed someone to address the problem. More often than not, these individuals are given the title of "chief wellness officer." My system's leaders weren't fond of the word "wellness," so we have a "chief clinician experience" officer—me.

It's an important role, though only a small part of my overall responsibilities. The role is broad—to put in place systems that promote the well-being of our physicians (There are separate initiatives for nurses and others.). I organized a hotline for physicians who may be having professional or personal difficulties and are seeking confidential help. I started a newsletter to promote the achievement of junior physician faculty members. I have put in place a peer support counseling program. And, yes, because I'm a writer, I started a writing group for physicians and other health care professionals. It's called "Words for Wellness," and its mission is to "learn, share, and grow through writing." We meet monthly for sessions that are a mix of basic instruction in writing skills, updates on writing projects, and brief exercises in response to writing prompts I have developed. Here is one example:

Select one of the three prompts below. Your task is to expand upon your selected prompt by 500 words or more. You will be asked to share your work with a peer and with the larger group at our next meeting.

1.   He didn't look anything like the monster I imagined. A man of roughly 60, slightly hunched over, and with a thin build and scruffy beard, it was difficult to imagine the terrible things he had done for which he was brought before us for his final appearance. He bore a resigned expression, even shrugging indifferently as he was asked if there was any anything he wished to say. The two burly guards went about their business professionally, strapping him down in a carefully rehearsed manner.

2.   Delayed. Canceled. Rescheduled. Weather. Maintenance. Crew shortage. All conspired to create airport chaos. Alex took it in stride, well equipped with tech paraphernalia to keep him occupied. He had a couple of granola bars in his carry-on bag which would have to do for dinner, since the lines at the airport eateries were so lengthy. A young woman sat across from him on the floor, her legs stretched out in front of her. She was listening to her phone through ear plugs. Like Alex, she seemed pretty comfortable. At one point Alex smiled and the young woman smiled back. Alex got up to toss out his granola bar wrappers and to buy a newspaper. When he returned the young woman was still there but sobbing uncontrollably.

3.   "Tell me why you think you're here, George," Dr. Bell asked.

"Aren't you supposed to tell me? It wasn't my idea, after all."

"I know why you're here. I want to see what your understanding is. Does that make sense?"

"It makes sense, but I still don't want to be here. I don't think I need to be here."

"I understand that," Dr. Bell said, "but just humor me for a bit. Tell me why you're here."

"OK, here it goes," George said as he took a deep breath. "I'm here because some people think I've said things that they believe are strange."

"That's certainly true, George. Let's explore that for a bit, shall we?"

I encourage you to try this exercise and hope you find it fun.

I find leading Words for Wellness immensely rewarding and enjoyable, and I would lead the group whether or not it was aligned with my hospital role or even if there was little evidence for the positive impact of creative writing on well-being. Fortunately, there is a small body of evidence in this area.

Lemay et al. at Yale have described the impact of a 2-day intensive workshop on writing narratives (see below) and found a positive impact on the ability to observe patients carefully and express empathy, as well as on their writing skills.[1] Though largely an opinion piece, Cronin et al. describe the benefits of creative writing in combatting professional burnout.[2] They note that Nobel Prize–winning neuroscientist and physician Santiago Ramón y Cajal used "fiction to take a vacation from the rules of scientific writing so that he could consider the future of science." Jay Baruch, in the *Journal of Medical Humanities*, describes how creative writing can promote both clinical excellence and empathy.[3] The evidence may be limited, and the small number of reports contain many anecdotes and opinions. This shouldn't be surprising: A rigorous study of the impact of writing on the well-being of biomedical professionals would require considerable resources, and, as you can imagine, such a study isn't a priority for many of the funding bodies mentioned throughout this book. Nevertheless, I think it's fair to say there's something there—a signal, a spark that strongly suggests that beyond the numerous academic benefits of writing, writing, especially in a mostly non-academic way, helps us cope with the many stressors of life. But how?

Cronin et al. write, "Although creative writing has generally produced positive results, no single theory adequately explains how or why. This can be attributed to the fact that expressive writing occurs on multiple levels . . . making a single explanatory theory unlikely." Hoyt et al. report in a randomized trial that emotional processing writing (in other words, writing about emotions related to a stressful or traumatic event) does have some benefit, especially when emotional processing is guided in a positive way, and more so for very stressful events.[4] The implications of their study for the kind of creative writing members of Words for Wellness engage in (we're working

[1] Lemay M, Encandela J, Sanders L, Reisman A. Writing well: The long-term effect on empathy, observation, and physician writing through a residency writers' workshop. J Grad Med Educ 2017Jun;9(3):357–360. doi:10.4300/JGME-D-16-00366.1. PMID: 28638517; PMCID: PMC5476388.

[2] Cronin M, Hubbard V, Cronin TA Jr, Frost P. Combatting professional burnout through creative writing. Clin Dermatol 2020 Sept–Oct;38(5):512–515. doi:10.1016/j.clindermatol.2020.05.004. Epub 2020 May 14. PMID: 33280794.

[3] Baruch JM. Creative writing as a medical instrument. J Med Humanit 2013;34:459–469.

[4] Hoyt MA, Darabos K, Llave K. Emotional processing writing and physiological stress responses: Understanding constructive and unconstructive processes. Cogn Emot 2021 Sept;35(6):1187–1194. doi:10.1080/02699931.2021.1929083. Epub 2021 May 20. PMID: 34011237.

on short stories as I write this chapter) are unclear. My own feeling is that all writing outside of the strictly scientific sphere is emotional. Expressing oneself in words on a page requires some processing of those emotions, and therefore might explain why at least a subset of biomedical professionals find creative writing both rewarding and stress-relieving.

So now that we've covered the why and potential how of writing for wellness, we should address what exactly you ought to consider writing. I suppose some of you might derive the same benefits from scientific writing that you or others might derive from writing essays, poetry, etc. But that isn't the case for most people. Scientific writing requires intense concentration and careful attention to the content, as well as more attention to the 5Cs, than creative writing, where you have more freedom to structure prose as you wish. You shouldn't completely abandon the 5Cs while pursuing creative writing, especially "commonness," which I discuss below. While it's undoubtedly rewarding in many ways, I don't think too many people find scientific writing effective in coping with the stressors of their lives. In fact, a requirement or obligation to write papers, grant applications, etc. is usually entwined with other professional responsibilities and can exert a heavy burden. In other words, scientific writing can be a source of rather than a treatment for stress. Cajal's description of fiction as a "vacation" from the "rules of scientific writing" is aligned with this idea. Scientific writing is the hard work; writing for wellness is the complementary leisure activity. There are no hard-and-fast rules, of course, about what to write. Words for Wellness participants have engaged in a number of projects, including personal essays, descriptions of patient illness, short stories, novels, and poetry. Whenever you explore non-scientific (for lack of a better term) writing in the biomedical professions, you're likely to encounter a few terms with which you should be familiar, since they encompass a great deal of the non-scientific writing activity of physicians and others.

You many have come across the term *medical humanities*. There are journals devoted to medical humanities and there are departments of medical humanities in many universities, usually as part of or closely affiliated with medical schools. Kirklin points out that there is no agreed-upon definition of medical humanities but provides the definition used by the Royal Free and University College Medical School in London: "Medical humanities is an interdisciplinary, and increasingly international endeavor that draws on the creative and intellectual strengths of diverse disciplines, including literature, art, creative writing, drama, film, music, philosophy, ethical decision making, anthropology, and history, in pursuit of medical educational goals."[5] This is a

---

[5] Kirklin D. The Center for Medical Humanities, Royal Free and University College Medical School, London, England. Acad Med 2003;78(10):1048–1053.

broad definition that encompasses not only writing but also many other creative forms. The key part of the definition is the educational intent. Through writing, music, etc., progress can be made in meeting goals in medical education, such as improving empathy and communication with patients. It's not hard to imagine, as an example, that reading about one patient's experience with cancer, either real or fictionalized, could promote empathy in medical students or other trainees. While at first glance it would appear that writing for wellness falls within the domain of medical humanities, there is no precise relationship between the two. I suppose some of you might choose to write about your own experiences with patients, or patient illness experiences, or some other aspect of your professional lives from which students or others could learn. But writing for wellness can encompass any topic of interest to the writer.

Another term you may have encountered is *narrative medicine*, sometimes referred to as *narrative-based medicine*. Zaharias points out that there is no standard accepted definition of the term,[6] though a committee of international experts defined narrative-based medicine as a "fundamental tool to acquire, comprehend, and integrate the different points of view of all the participants having a role in the illness experience."[7] I believe somewhat abstract definitions like these do a disservice to those of us who are genuinely interested in learning more and perhaps applying our interests in writing to the field. Essentially, almost all definitions of narrative or narrative-based medicine encompass the use of patient stories to better understand the experience of illness. This is something I know a little about. My first book, *Primary Care Management: Cases and Discussions*,[8] includes a series of chapters on the most common problems in primary care. Each chapter begins with a detailed story of a patient's life. After the story, the patient's actual medical concerns are presented and the course of the illness is described gradually, as the learner or reader contemplates the next step in diagnosis, evaluation, and management. The chapters are accompanied by detailed, evidence-based (for the time) recommendations. At the time, I didn't know I was practicing or teaching narrative medicine by writing the book. My fundamental assumption was that by understanding a patient's life, as a physician, I could better manage his or her illness. The life stories in the book are entirely fictional. Writing them

⁶ Zaharias G. What is narrative-based medicine? Narrative-based medicine 1. Can Fam Physician 2018;64(3):176–180. PMID: 29540381; PMCID: PMC5851389.

⁷ Fioretti C, Mazzocco K, Riva S, et al. Research studies on patients' illness experience using the narrative medicine approach: A systematic review. BMJ Open 2016;6(7):e011220. doi:10.1136/bmjopen-2016-011220. PMID: 27417197; PMCID: PMC4947803.

⁸ Rao G. *Primary care management: Cases and discussions*. Sage, 1999.

was immensely enjoyable. In fact, the life stories and the illness course and medical recommendations in the book complement each other. So, I was balancing my scientific writing with fiction, much like Cajal.

A final term you may have heard of is *expressive writing*. Expressive writing has been defined as "a tool through which the subject describes his/her most profound thoughts and feelings about emotional events."[9] The study by Hoyt et al. mentioned above described the positive benefits of emotional processing writing, which is another way of saying expressive writing. Tonarelli et al. report the benefit of expressive writing, compared to neutral writing, in terms of dealing with negative thoughts over the course of writing sessions.[10]

I've described these concepts not for their practical value, but because you are likely to encounter them and may wonder what exactly they mean. The whole idea of writing for wellness is gradually gaining traction. The University of Arizona hosts a conference annually on the subject, at which I spoke in 2024.[11] This is a science and a movement that is still in its infancy, so it's not surprising that the terms, concepts, and evidence base for the benefits of writing for wellness are still in development. What I can offer are some concrete lessons and resources from Words for Wellness.

First, let's discuss the motivation for members of Words for Wellness to participate. It is true that writing, in particular creative writing, has some benefit in terms of coping with stress and promoting wellness. I don't believe, however, that's enough to inspire participation in a group. Imagine you are a physician or other biomedical professional who, after a long, difficult day at work, is offered a chance to do some creative writing, with guidance, to help you cope with the stress you face. I think most people in that situation, me included, would simply rather just go home and relax, or pursue another activity that doesn't require as much concentration and effort. The therapeutic value of writing may be real, but it still takes a great deal of effort, and motivating busy professionals to take part for a potential therapeutic value is likely to be difficult. Instead, in our group, we focus on goals for writing. Some members want to learn to write well so that they can apply new and refined skills to projects they have in mind. Others come with projects in development they would like to advance for publication. Others simply enjoy the camaraderie of the group and express a strong interest in learning about writing and about

[9] Tonarelli A, Cosentino C, Artioli D, et al. Expressive writing: A tool to help health workers: Research project on the benefits of expressive writing. Acta Biomed 2017 Nov 30;88(5S):13–21. doi:10.23750/abm.v88i5-S.6877. PMID: 29189701; PMCID: PMC6357577.

[10] Tonarelli A, Cosentino C, Artioli D, et al. Expressive writing: A tool to help health workers: Research project on the benefits of expressive writing. Acta Biomed 2017 Nov 30;88(5S):13–21. doi:10.23750/abm.v88i5-S.6877. PMID: 29189701; PMCID: PMC6357577.

[11] https://writingandwellbeing.arizona.edu/. Accessed July 27, 2024.

others' writing. Many have more than one motivation. What is common is that they want to achieve something tangible. We are highly driven health care professionals, after all, and that usually means publication. It means, for example, having a short story published in a literary journal and then sharing the story widely. The sense of satisfaction our members feel from such accomplishments is immense.

Second, let's talk about skills. Writing of any kind, as you, a reader of this book, have undoubtedly concluded, is not easy. The great English novelist, playwright, and short story writer Somerset Maugham, who was also a qualified physician, is said to have encountered a surgeon who told him, "When I retire, I want to write novels like you." Maugham responded humorously, "When I retire, I want to practice surgery." Some believe the encounter never really happened and that the humorous exchange is just an "urban legend." My point, however, is that as difficult as creative writing actually is, many, many people assume that it's straightforward and easy. All you need is a good idea for a story (and most people assume they have one), and then a computer or pen and paper, and you're all set. Then, when you finish your fantastic novel, you will sell thousands of copies and become rich. Wrong!

In an essay in the *New York Times* Joseph Epstein points out that 81% of Americans feel they should write a book.[12] I have always been surprised by such statistics. After all, I doubt a high percentage of Americans feel they should compose a symphony or paint a landscape. For some reason, writing is perceived as a relatively easy activity—perhaps because we've all written something fairly substantial at one point in our lives, even if it's for a school assignment or college admission essay. The sad fact is that, assuming someone is disciplined enough to write a book, getting it published in some form or another (e.g., self-publishing, online publishing, vanity presses [publishers you pay to publish your book]) is relatively easy, so the number of books available has grown hugely in recent years. Epstein wrote more than 20 years ago, "Why should so many people think they can write a book, especially at a time when so many people who actually do write books turn out not really to have a book in them—or at least not one that many other people can be made to care about?" There are simply too many books and not enough readers. That doesn't mean that you shouldn't try to get your creative writing published. We need new things to read just like we need new songs to listen to. But be prepared for lots of rejections. If publication is the goal, perseverance is necessary, along with necessary skills. Just as you can't simply play a musical instrument

---

[12] https://www.nytimes.com/2002/09/28/opinion/think-you-have-a-book-in-you-think-again.html. Accessed July 27, 2024.

(at least in a way anyone would want to listen to) without training, you can't write creatively without some training.

I have found it astonishing that many highly educated professionals, some of whom are skillful scientific writers, can't write a decent story. Let's forget about grammar, punctuation, and spelling, since there are lots of software programs around to correct problems with those. Coming up with an idea for a story is relatively easy; anyone who has lived usually has something interesting to share. Making it coherent and believable is another matter. I believe a lot of biomedical professionals haven't done any creative writing since they were children. Sadly, sometimes their skills are stuck—if not in childhood, certainly in adolescence. Words for Wellness is not just a forum to share writing and advance writing projects. The more important goal of the group is to learn creative writing skills. The general consensus is that creative writing can be taught, though there are lots of opinions as to the best way to do so.[13] There is a field of "creative writing studies" and an associated journal.[14] Much of the pedagogical tradition of creative writing is intense and time-consuming (e.g., the famous Iowa workshops) and simply impractical for busy biomedical professionals. I've adopted a much simpler approach for Words for Wellness.

We review the 5Cs, which, though intended for scientific writing, are certainly applicable to some extent to creative writing as well. In particular, as I noted earlier, "commonness," the avoidance of fancy words and flowery language, is important. Fancy words fill the pages of new creative writers: How something sounds while they read it is mistakenly thought of as a sign of both creativity and sophistication. Instead, I insist our members follow Hemingway's advice to use simple language and short sentences and paragraphs.[15] Simplicity and conciseness are elegant. Using a word or words in ways they were not intended to be used is a common problem, so we spend a great deal of time on correct usage. After several lessons, members of our group are encouraged to complete an online quiz I designed.

Most importantly, rather than recreating the wheel with new materials, I insist that all members read Benjamin Dryer's *Dreyer's English: An Utterly Correct Guide to Clarity and Style*.[16] It will take you no more than a few days to read at a leisurely pace. It's brilliant. It's funny. It will provide you with important skills you need before you start creative writing. Most importantly, it will raise your consciousness of what you are writing as you write, so that you

---

[13] Vanderslice S, Manery R (eds.). *Can creative writing really be taught: Resisting lore in creative writing pedagogy* (10th anniversary edition). Bloomsbury Academic, 2017.
[14] https://repository.rit.edu/jcws/. Accessed July 27, 2024.
[15] https://www.wordsthatsing.com.au/post/hemingway-rules. Accessed July 28, 2024.
[16] Dreyer B. *Dreyer's English: An utterly correct guide to clarity and style*. Random House, 2019.

consciously avoid using flowery language and incoherent gibberish. It will also help you pass my usage quiz.

Once we've discussed each member's goals, covered essential skills through presentations and exercises I've developed, and read *Dreyer's English*, we tackle prompts like the one above and more ambitious writing projects for publication.

In summary, I encourage all of you not only to improve your scientific writing but also to explore writing for wellness as a valuable, complementary activity. While I can't guarantee you will find it enjoyable and rewarding, there is no harm in trying.

15

What About AI?

See if you can go a day without hearing something about "artificial intelligence" (or, much more likely, the simple acronym "AI") on TV, at work, or elsewhere. I can't remember a day free from hearing "AI" over the past year. AI is seemingly everywhere, and its potential is said to be limitless. My first knowledge of anything that resembles AI was when watching the old Stanley Kubrick movie *2001: A Space Odyssey*, which featured H.A.L. (Heuristically Programmed Algorithmic Computer). H.A.L is an AI device and a reliable member of the crew of the spaceship *Discovery*. At some point, H.A.L. starts making mistakes, and members of the crew decide to shut him down. H.A.L. is a sentient being who can play chess, recognize faces, and carry out complex tasks like many computers today, but he also has feelings. Feeling threatened, H.A.L. decides to kill the astronauts who plan to shut him down. The film came out in 1968, and in it, H.A.L. was created in 1992. It is now nearly 35 years after the time in which the movie is set, and we are nowhere near developing machines that can truly think for themselves, let alone have feelings on which they act.

What we *do* have is machine learning that relies on analysis of huge amounts of data to recognize patterns and generate output based on statistical inference. This itself is no small feat and is one that, as many have insisted, has the potential to transform many aspects of human life.

While discussing the possibility of writing this book, a colleague told me that he didn't think it would serve an important need, as AI could be used to write papers and grants. Scientific writing skills, in his view, would be obsolete. As someone who teaches writing skills, that's indeed a grim prospect.

Let's consider what generative (i.e., able to generate new material) AI can do. I asked ChatGPT to write a narrative review article about best practices for diagnosis of dementia in primary care. Here's the first part of what it came up with:

Narrative Review: Best Practices for the Diagnosis of Dementia in Primary Care
Abstract
Dementia is a growing public health concern, with significant implications for patients, caregivers, and healthcare systems. Early and accurate diagnosis

in primary care settings is crucial for optimal management and improved outcomes. This review aims to synthesize current best practices for the diagnosis of dementia in primary care, emphasizing the importance of early recognition, appropriate use of diagnostic tools, and the integration of multidisciplinary care.

Introduction

Dementia is a syndrome characterized by a decline in cognitive function beyond what might be expected from normal aging, impacting daily living activities. Alzheimer's disease (AD) is the most common cause, but other types include vascular dementia, Lewy body dementia, and frontotemporal dementia. With the aging global population, the prevalence of dementia is expected to rise, making early diagnosis in primary care crucial.

Primary care physicians (PCPs) are often the first point of contact for patients with cognitive concerns. Early recognition of dementia allows for timely interventions that can improve quality of life, delay progression, and provide patients and caregivers with essential support. However, diagnosing dementia in primary care can be challenging due to the subtlety of early symptoms, time constraints, and the overlap with other conditions such as depression or delirium.

Early Recognition and Screening

Early recognition of dementia begins with awareness of its risk factors and symptoms. Patients over 65, especially those with a family history of dementia, cardiovascular risk factors, or previous cognitive complaints, should be monitored closely. PCPs should be vigilant for early signs, such as memory complaints, changes in behavior or personality, and difficulties with language, reasoning, or daily tasks.

Screening Tools: *While routine screening of asymptomatic individuals is not universally recommended, targeted cognitive screening is crucial for those presenting with memory concerns or other cognitive symptoms. Commonly used tools in primary care include:*

- *Mini-Mental State Examination (MMSE): A 30-point questionnaire assessing orientation, recall, attention, calculation, language, and visual-spatial skills.*
- *Montreal Cognitive Assessment (MoCA): A 30-point test more sensitive for detecting mild cognitive impairment, covering executive functions, memory, attention, language, and orientation.*

- *General Practitioner Assessment of Cognition (GPCOG): Combines patient assessment with an informant interview, focusing on recent cognitive decline.*

These tools provide an initial assessment but are not definitive diagnostic instruments. A positive screen should prompt further evaluation or referral to a specialist.

What do you think? I think it's an impressive beginning. The writing is excellent, and the content, while a bit too general to be useful in my view, is certainly appropriate and accurate. Had I given ChatGPT more specific instructions, such as "Write a narrative review suitable for the journal *American Family Physician*" or "Write a narrative review summarizing developments in the primary care diagnosis of dementia over the past 5 years," the content might be a bit more useful.

What if someone provided those instructions and an AI program created an entire manuscript that was then submitted to a journal? As the editor of Oxford University Press's *Family Practice*, not knowing I was reading an AI-generated article, I might be impressed enough for the submission to send it out for peer review. Reviewers might like it as well, and it could get published bearing the names of authors who did virtually nothing to create it. To say that this raises serious ethical questions is an understatement.

The ethical issues involved with AI and scientific publication have yet to be resolved, since the technology became mainstream so recently and so quickly. OpenAI's ChatGPT is the fastest-adopted technology in human history.[1]

The field of AI, as machine learning and other forms, is moving so fast that the content of this chapter may be obsolete shortly after it is published. Nevertheless, I'll do my best to tell you what I know and what I believe about the use of AI in scientific writing.

First, let's clarify what exactly we're talking about. We're talking about the use of AI to write papers. AI can be used for other aspects of research, of course. For example, AI might be used to design a clinical trial. In other cases, AI itself might be the subject of research. New electronic health record systems, for example, feature AI tools with which patients can interact. One or more of these might become the subject for a research study and a paper. In the context of scientific publication, some journal or grant reviewers might be tempted to use AI for peer review. For example, a reviewer might cut and paste the entire

[1] https://arstechnica.com/information-technology/2023/02/chatgpt-sets-record-for-fastest-growing-user-base-in-history-report-says/. Accessed August 29, 2024.

contents of a paper and ask ChatGPT or another AI tool to assess its quality. There is no journal or other scientific body that allows this sort of use of AI. The rationale is quite simple—As a peer reviewer, you are required to keep the content of materials to be reviewed confidential. By cutting and pasting it into an AI tool, you are sharing it externally, which breaches that confidentiality.

Can AI actually be used to write a paper? I provided the example above to demonstrate the impressive (if a little frightening) capabilities of generative AI in creating a paper from scratch. But that's not how many researchers would likely use AI. Instead, they may enter some details, such as an abstract presented at a conference or even some raw data, and then ask an AI tool to construct an entire paper based on this input. This would, of course, make things much easier for those with poor writing skills, or those whose first language is not the language in which they wish to publish.

At the time of writing this chapter (September 2024) publishers, journals, and associations have adopted some general policies about the use of AI that are worth reviewing. In general, the use of AI is permitted under certain conditions. Ganjavi et al. have reviewed publishers' and journals' instructions for the use of generative AI for writing papers in a paper published in the *British Medical Journal* in November 2023.[2] Their goal was to identify commonalities among various organizations. In addition to publishers and journals, they review general policies from the Committee on Publication Ethics (COPE), whose members include representatives from journals, publishers, universities and research institutes, and the World Association of Medical Editors (WAME). Ganjavi et al. point out that there is significant heterogeneity in instructions. Two of the world's most prestigious journals have restrictive policies about using AI to write papers: *Science* explicitly prohibits it; *Lancet* limits AI to use in improving the "readability and language of the work." Tools to improve readability and language, as you've undoubtedly discovered, are available within word processing tools such as Microsoft Word or in freestanding programs such as Grammarly.

There are two aspects of policy that are uniform across various organizations:

1. An AI tool cannot be listed as an author, as it cannot assume responsibility for the work. All authors must assume responsibility for what they wish to have published when they use AI.

---

[2] Ganjavi C, Eppler MB, Pekcan A, et al. Publishers' and journals' instructions to authors on use of generative artificial intelligence in academic and scientific publishing: Bibliometric analysis. BMJ 2024;384:e077192. doi:10.1136/bmj-2023-077192. PMID: 38296328; PMCID: PMC10828852.

2. Use of AI requires detailed disclosure, including in what sections it was used; the specific AI program, manufacturer, and version; and dates used.

Ganjavi et al. point out that there are some inconsistencies in policies. Some of these I would view as relatively minor (e.g., in what part of the paper an AI disclosure should be made, and different terms for "disclose," such as "report" or "note"). They also note that policies have been developed internally by organizations with no identifiable systematic consensus development process. This of course isn't unexpected, given the speed with which the technology has emerged.

To address the problem of heterogeneity in policies, Dr. Giovanni Cacciamani (a co-author of the Ganjavi et al. paper) has started an initiative to systematically develop guidelines: the ChatGPT, Generative Artificial Intelligence and Natural Large Language models for Accountable Reporting and Use (CANGARU) guidelines.[3] The guideline development process they describe in their protocol is expansive and includes the bibliometric analysis that formed the basis for the Ganjavi et al. paper as well as multiple Delphi survey rounds, a consensus meeting, piloting of guidelines, etc.

While all this attention to methodology is impressive, I think it's overkill. It will take considerable time for CANGARU to fulfill its objectives, and, by that point, the technology may have evolved to a point where the guidelines are obsolete. Also, I believe the two requirements for the use of AI in writing—not listing an AI program as an author and disclosing its use in whatever details are requested—are likely to remain the standard across multiple organizations. How these two requirements are met may continue to vary despite the availability of consensus-driven guidelines.

The *Journal of the American Medical Association* (JAMA) and the family of JAMA journals has a relatively straightforward way for authors to address the two requirements.[4] Authors are first asked:

Did you use AI, a language model, machine learning, or similar technologies to create or assist with creation or editing of any of the content in this submission (e.g., text, tables, figures, video)? (Note: this does not include basic tools for checking grammar, spelling, references, etc.)

[3] https://arxiv.org/abs/2307.08974. Accessed August 28, 2024.
[4] Flanagin A, Kendall-Taylor J, Bibbins-Domingo K. Guidance for authors, peer reviewers, and editors on use of AI, language models, and chatbots. JAMA 2023 Aug 22;330(8):702–703. doi:10.1001/jama.2023.12500. PMID: 37498593.

A "yes" response prompts the following questions:

Please provide a description of the AI-generated content that is included in this submission and the name of the model or tool used, version and extension numbers, and manufacturer in the space below.

Please confirm that you take responsibility for the integrity of the content generated by these tools and that you have provided a description of such generated content and the name of the model or tool used, version and extension numbers, and manufacturer in the Acknowledgment or Methods section of the manuscript.

Something similar to this approach can be found on many journals' and publishers' websites.

All this having been said, I think there is a much bigger question to address. While AI might have a valuable role in literature reviews, the conduct of research, and even planning for publication or grant submissions, should you actually use it to help write?

As the author of a book on scientific writing, I obviously believe scientific writing skills are important and will remain important. I don't think scientific writing skills will become obsolete anytime soon. Consider this analogy: There are lots of powerful statistical programs out there, but also plenty of jobs for biostatisticians who can help design research and analyze results. Their expertise is still considered necessary. Someone with no statistical expertise is ill advised to start entering results into a statistical program hoping for a useful and valid analysis. At this time, AI is prone to inaccuracy and bias, though that situation is likely to get better in coming years. However AI is used, you must carefully review the output if you are submitting a paper to a journal or an application to a granting body.

The issue of policy and the ongoing and future need to write well are two issues. My own thinking is that writing a paper, an abstract, or a grant application is *an integral part of the scientific process.* You cannot write a paper as fast as ChatGPT; you have to think carefully about what content to include, including what results are most important and what pitfalls you encountered. This thinking process is part of what it means to be a scientist, in my opinion. And since writing is part of the science, just as science is part of the writing, I would encourage you to use AI cautiously for writing. When you assume responsibility for written scientific work, the assumption is that you have conceived it, organized it, written it, and reviewed it. I believe these tasks are part of, rather than distinct from, the entire research process.

In a year or two, my thoughts may be less relevant. Policies and guidelines may change. Some people (not me) even believe AI is a passing fad. Let's all stay tuned to see what happens.

16
Giving Feedback to Others

This book is all about writing, and while throughout I've recommended seeking feedback from others about your writing, especially to improve clarity, to this point I haven't discussed giving feedback. While writing may be a solitary activity, carried out in settings where you can't be distracted, writers themselves are often and should be part of a larger community. I encourage you to join the Biomedical Writer's Handbook Community online. There you will find more opportunities to practice, learn about writing opportunities, get tips to improve your writing, and receive updates on developments in the field, such as advancements in AI. I believe giving feedback to others about their writing is an integral part of being a biomedical writer for a few compelling reasons:

1. Just like reading lots of scientific papers is likely to improve your writing as you become more familiar with how to express ideas clearly or what forms different types of articles should take, reading the writing of those who solicit your feedback will help you learn new ways to write better.
2. The second reason why providing feedback is vital involves the principle of reciprocity. You will undoubtedly need feedback from others. In fact, I can't imagine submitting an article to a journal without seeking feedback from at least one of my peers. They in turn are comfortable seeking my feedback. So we both benefit, and not offering feedback really isn't an option.
3. Providing constructive feedback is inherently satisfying. You're helping someone else. You're influencing how they express their work. You feel honored that they value your suggestions.

If giving feedback is part of what it means to be a writer, knowing best practices for doing so is really important. Feedback that consists of nothing but praise is meaningless and unhelpful. On the other hand, feedback that is overly harsh may discourage the writer and will likely cause him or her to stop seeking your feedback in the future. Rather than thinking about "a happy medium," it's best to go about giving feedback systematically, with the end goal of helping someone improve their work.

As you can imagine, there is neither a well-researched approach to giving feedback to others nor any consensus on how to do so. What I recommend is based on my many years of writing, editing, and seeking and delivering feedback. There are some published recommendations upon which I've partly based what you'll find below.[1] We use this approach in Words for Wellness, and it has worked very well.

First, when your feedback is solicited, *ask what feedback is desired*. Start by asking the writer what specifically he or she would like feedback about. If the writer is unsure, offer some suggestions, such as:

> "Are you worried something isn't clear?"
> "Would you like me to read over your significance section to see if I believe it offers a compelling rationale for the research?"

A novice might be very tentative or unsure about what to ask. For novice writers, it's also fine to ask,

> "What section do you believe is the strongest?"
> "Which section do you believe still needs work?"

Notice the gentle, constructive language in these questions. Writing in any form is deeply personal, since the writer has invested heavily in the end product. Always be respectful to the writer no matter his or her level of experience.

Second, *don't worry about typos, grammar, or punctuation*. Problems with these areas don't appear in this book for a reason: There are lots of ways to correct them before a piece is submitted for publication. Spelling and grammar check features in word processing programs such as Microsoft Word can be applied to a piece anytime. Checking a piece for spelling and grammar errors isn't the best use of your time as someone giving feedback. If you get too caught up in such minor issues, you might also lose sight of more important ones, such as problems with the coherence of a manuscript or grant application. It's also unlikely that someone soliciting your feedback is looking for a spell-check from you.

Third, *always give feedback about the piece, not about the writer*. For instance, telling the writer "You tend to use flowery language" could be deeply hurtful, even if you have become familiar with the writer's work and your observation is actually true. Remember, we want writers to keep writing and to

---

[1] Watling C, Lingard L. Giving feedback on others' writing. Perspect Med Educ 2019;8:25–27.

learn how to write better. Sure, this comment may inspire the writer to avoid such language—or it could discourage him from writing at all, which certainly isn't the objective of your feedback. Saying instead "I believe this sentence could be stated more simply" is more constructive.

Here's another example of less-constructive feedback from creative writing: "As I read this, your train of thought is awfully hard to follow." A better alternative might be "I'm a bit confused by these paragraphs. In the first, the lead character is a little girl. In the next, she's all grown up." You might think the first sentence is relatively benign, and in fact many writers may find it helpful. Some, however, may be offended: "Is he saying I'm a scatterbrain?!" The second sentence is not only more neutral but also specifies what exactly was confusing. You should adhere to the same principle when delivering feedback about scientific writing: Be specific and don't imply that there is something wrong with the writer's thought process. Instead of simply labeling a paragraph as "confusing," for example, specify exactly what you don't understand. This gives the writer the best opportunity to correct the problem.

My final bits of advice deal with the logistics of delivering feedback and its format. Assuming you are willing to provide feedback and the writer is enthusiastic about receiving it, make sure you *confirm up front by what date the writer needs the feedback.* Many biomedical writers, novices especially, seek feedback a few days before a manuscript, abstract, or grant application is due. This is problematic for a couple of reasons:

1. If something is due so soon and you are able to give valuable feedback, the writer may need to make extensive revisions without enough time.
2. Feedback that is needed in a couple of days is unlikely to represent your best or most thorough work. For a full grant application, manuscript, or other scientific work, I recommend at least 2 full weeks. If you choose to read and comment on the work in one sitting, this allows you to set aside the few hours needed. Alternatively, you can work on feedback in short sessions over the course of the 2 weeks.

For most biomedical works, writers seek feedback that is very specific, with comments and suggested edits added to a piece in Microsoft Word or other program. This is perfectly reasonable and acceptable. However, I also recommend that you *provide an overview paragraph,* either on the manuscript (typically in electronic form) or in an email. An overview paragraph allows you to highlight general concerns and strengths of the piece that may be lost if the writer dives right into your specific feedback. The paragraph need not be long (perhaps 100 to 200 words) and could give the writer an idea of what more specific feedback to look for. Here's an example:

> *Hi Mindy:*
> *Thanks for allowing me to look over your grant application. I learned a great deal about the management of venomous snake bites in remote areas. Please see the attached version of your manuscript for my specific feedback, with suggested edits and comments.*
>
> *I do have two general concerns. I am concerned that your second aim is contingent upon your first. If your team is unable to produce enough anti-venom, will it really matter if there are facilities to which it can be delivered? My second major concern is that reviewers will see the problem as one of misadventures among a small group of reckless people, rather than a significant public health problem. Rather than improving the distribution of anti-venom, reviewers might suggest preventive measures such as education about not disturbing snakes or wearing protective clothing. How would you respond to such criticism?*
>
> *All things considered, I think your application has a lot of potential and I look forward to hearing about it getting funded!*

The reviewer uses a respectful tone and begins with thanking the writer for the feedback opportunity. This is the sort of tone that promotes reciprocity and community. Notice how the two major concerns are phrased. "I am concerned that your second aim is contingent upon" rather than "Your second aim depends on successfully meeting the first, and that just won't fly!" The reviewer phrases the second concern as a potential problem for those who will be reading the proposal, regardless of what the person delivering feedback believes. Finally, the reviewer ends with a positive statement. This is very important as it provides the needed encouragement for the writer to take the feedback seriously and to make the recommended changes.

A final issue that sometimes comes up is whether or not you should provide a second or even third round of feedback. In most cases, *don't provide another round of feedback.* I discourage this since it takes up so much time. The exception is those whom you are mentoring. My mentees over the years have received multiple rounds of feedback, and hopefully have learned a little bit each time. In the spirit of community and reciprocity, one round of feedback should suffice. The writer may be seeking feedback from more than one person. It's up to the writer to consider all the feedback carefully and put his or her best work forward. Too many rounds of feedback can actually be prob-lematic. The writer may believe he or she has incorporated your suggestions adequately, but you may feel differently. You may also feel compelled to note minor problems you didn't notice the first time, and this can be discouraging to the writer. So, with few exceptions, stick to one round.

17

A Few Words on Collaborative Writing

As I've told you before, the best way for you to write, in my opinion, is alone in a quiet place. That applies to any sort of writing. Curiously, you'll find lots of writing groups (mostly for creative writing) for people who want to get together, sometimes to discuss their writing, but also sometimes to write together. There is a group called "Shut Up and Write!" (www.shutupwrite.com) whose members benefit from the collective discipline and motivation of a group to meet in a coffee shop or someplace similar and buckle down to write for an hour or two. I'm skeptical of the value of these sorts of activities. Writing in a group might provide some collective discipline, but if you lack the discipline to write alone, group writing may also disintegrate into nothing more than a social gathering.

That having been said, when it comes to scientific writing, the vast majority of works are written by more than person. Papers with dozens of authors aren't uncommon. So, writing as a group, or collaboratively, even if individual segments are written alone, is quite normal.

There are some published recommendations for collaborative writing. Some of these deal with the use of various cloud-based tools to collaborate on writing projects (e.g. Google Docs).[1] Others discuss being inclusive, delivering feedback, and setting expectations for members. There are different specific strategies for writing a paper together. Lingard provides a categorization of common strategies:[2]

- *One for all*: One author does all the writing and solicits feedback and edits from the others.
- *Each in sequence*: Different authors complete parts of a paper in sequence. One author writes the introduction; the next writes the methods section, etc.
- *All in parallel*: The paper is divided into parts and then each group member drafts each part. The parts are then collectively revised. Thus, everyone is working on an introduction, for example, at the same time.

---

[1] Yilmaz Y, Gottlieb M, Haas MRC, et al. Remote collaborative writing: A guide to writing within a virtual community of practice. J Grad Med Educ 2022 Jun;14(3):256–259. doi:10.4300/JGME-D-21-01108.1. Epub 2022 Jun 13. PMID: 35754624; PMCID: PMC9200254.

[2] Lingard L. Collaborative writing: Strategies and activities for writing productively together. Perspect Med Educ 2021 Jun;10(3):163–166. doi:10.1007/s40037-021-00668-7. Epub 2021 May 7. PMID: 33961205; PMCID: PMC8187494.

- *All in reaction*: The document is created collectively in real time and individual members adjust to each other's edits and changes almost immediately.
- *Multimodal*: This involves the use of multiple strategies.

Much of what is written about how to write collaboratively suggests that there is a finite set of principles and strategies that have proven to be effective in different circumstances. I don't believe this is true. Collaborative writing is often a fluid process, with different strategies adopted at different points to get a manuscript across the finish line. It also depends greatly upon the composition of the writing group, especially in terms of the members' experience both in writing and in collaborating in the past. I believe that choosing a specific strategy such as "All in reaction" or an online collaboration platform is far less important than having a motivated team in which each member contributes in the best way he or she can.

I'm not going to give you "10 simple rules" for collaborative writing.[3] What I *can* offer are a few lessons I've learned in organizing and leading collaborative writing teams. My most relevant experience comes from my past role as Chair of the American Heart Association (AHA)'s Obesity Committee. The AHA is an influential organization that issues scientific statements and guidelines on timely topics in cardiovascular prevention and treatment. The preparation process for these scientific statements is typically led by an experienced scientist, after a significant approval process. Teams are assembled that reflect experience, expertise, and the diversity of the AHA's membership and biomedical workforce. It's important to include inexperienced authors, for example, as well as scientists from underrepresented minority backgrounds. It's been my privilege to lead several of these teams[4,5,6] and to have participated

---

[3] Frassl MA, Hamilton DP, Denfeld BA, et al. Ten simple rules for collaboratively writing a multi-authored paper. PLoS Comput Biol 2018 Nov 15;14(11):e1006508. doi:10.1371/journal.pcbi.1006508. PMID: 30439938; PMCID: PMC6237291.

[4] Rao G, Lopez-Jimenez F, Boyd J, et al; American Heart Association Council on Lifestyle and Cardiometabolic Health; Council on Cardiovascular and Stroke Nursing; Council on Cardiovascular Surgery and Anesthesia; Council on Clinical Cardiology; Council on Functional Genomics and Translational Biology; and Stroke Council. Methodological standards for meta-analyses and qualitative systematic reviews of cardiac prevention and treatment studies: A scientific statement from the American Heart Association. Circulation 2017 Sep 5;136(10):e172–e194. doi:10.1161/CIR.0000000000000523. Epub 2017 Aug 7. PMID: 28784624.

[5] Rao G, Powell-Wiley TM, Ancheta I, et al; American Heart Association Obesity Committee of the Council on Lifestyle and Cardiometabolic Health. Identification of obesity and cardiovascular risk in ethnically and racially diverse populations: A scientific statement from the American Heart Association. Circulation 2015 Aug 4;132(5):457–72. doi:10.1161/CIR.0000000000000223. Epub 2015 Jul 6. Erratum in: Circulation 2015 Aug 25;132(8):e130. doi:10.1161/CIR.0000000000000291. PMID: 26149446.

[6] Rao G, Burke LE, Spring BJ, et al; American Heart Association Obesity Committee of the Council on Nutrition, Physical Activity and Metabolism; Council on Clinical Cardiology; Council on Cardiovascular

as a member of several more. Though you'll find the lessons below in similar forms in other places. I think these are the most important things to keep in mind, rather than worrying about which cloud-based platform to use to share versions of a document versus simply emailing versions back and forth.

1. *It takes leadership.* Let's assume you have participated in a research project that has just concluded, and it's time to write a paper based on the results. The paper will never materialize unless someone leads the effort. The leader is often the principal investigator of the project, but it could also be a junior co-investigator. What matters is that the individual moves the writing forward with clear assignments as to what parts each member of the team is to complete, by what deadline, etc. The leader should establish the order of authorship based on overall contributions to the project (including writing the paper). The leaders should pull all the sections of a paper together to make sure they are coherent and follow a consistent style. A paper moves forward through regular meetings where progress is discussed and nudges are given to individual authors to complete their sections. Feedback should follow the recommendations in Chapter 16. Without a leader, the collaborative effort becomes a mess as individual writers work on the paper haphazardly, or the effort doesn't get started at all.

2. *Writing group members vary vastly in their experience and writing ability.* Differences in experience and writing ability are inevitable among biomedical research teams. Your team may include people who've basically never written anything beyond basic communications related to the project and others whose first language is not English. You should keep this in mind up front to avoid getting frustrated. Instead, pair more experienced writers with less experienced ones. Experienced authors can serve as coaches and help others revise their work before it is presented to the larger group. It's not reasonable to assign, say, the methods section to an inexperienced author without coaching.

3. *Deadlines are critically important.* A writing team works toward a common goal. If one or more members miss a deadline, it puts the entire project as risk. This is especially true when deadlines are determined externally—for example, when a grant application is due on a certain

Nursing; Council on the Kidney in Cardiovascular Disease; Stroke Council. New and emerging weight management strategies for busy ambulatory settings: A scientific statement from the American Heart Association endorsed by the Society of Behavioral Medicine. Circulation 2011 Sep 6;124(10):1182–203. doi:10.1161/CIR.0b013e31822b9543. Epub 2011 Aug 8. PMID: 21824925.

date. There is no magic formula to helping your team meet deadlines beyond making sure that the deadlines are realistic and that everyone understands their importance. Many teams in the biomedical disciplines are transitory—post-docs leave for new positions, senior scientists retire, etc. Missed deadlines and delayed projects will decrease the probability that the writing project will ever be finished.

4. *The rewards of collaborative writing are substantial.* I've gone solo for much of my writing, but collaborating on papers has been one of the activities I've found most rewarding. My first major effort leading a large team was a contribution to the Rational Clinical Exam series in the *Journal of the American Medical Association* (JAMA) on Parkinson disease.[7] We met often over the course of a year to discuss research progress and worked diligently on specific sections. Progress meetings were often held over coffee, lunch, or dinner. Several of the team members were inexperienced writers at that time but continued to write and to grow as academicians. We all valued the experience, not only because the end product was a high-profile publication but also because it was simply a lot of fun.

[7] Rao G, Fisch L, Srinivasan S, et al. Does this patient have Parkinson disease? JAMA 2003 Jan 15;289(3):347–353. doi:10.1001/jama.289.3.347. PMID: 12525236.

18

Ten Practice Problems

You've nearly made it to the end, and I hope the book has been helpful so far. Coming this far has hopefully helped you learn how to become a better biomedical writer. To actually become a better biomedical writer, though, requires practice, and lots of it. In my nearly 30 years of writing and editing scientific prose of some sort or another, I can tell you that for me no amount of learning theory, taking courses on writing papers and grant proposals, or reading books on writing was *nearly* as helpful as lots and lots of practice. As I noted, writing daily is a good habit for those starting out, even if it's not necessary later on. I write daily, partly out of necessity and partly because I enjoy it. You may already have one or more projects lined up that will give you practice. In any case, I think you can benefit from completing the 10 exercises that follow.

The purpose of the exercises is two-fold. First, I want you to be able to assess how much you've learned in this book. If an exercise seems too difficult, review the relevant part of the book. Second, I want to give you simple opportunities to improve.

The exercises are organized according to the most common writing tasks we've covered. As always, pay close attention to the 5Cs as you complete them. I hope you find this chapter helpful.

Exercise #1

Rewrite this short introduction to a paper so that it follows a more logical order and is more concise:

Our goal was to compare an artificial intelligence (AI)-supported system for interpretation of mammography screening results to a standard, current practice of double reading by radiologists for the identification of breast cancer. Breast cancer is a significant public health problem and screening mammography is effective and recommended for detection of early cancerous lesions. Interpretation of screening mammograms is associated with a significant

workload for radiologists, and is also prone to inaccuracy in the form of missed
cancers. AI has shown significant promise in identifying suspicious lesions in
other types of radiological investigations such as thoracic imaging and brain
imaging. Its usefulness in screening mammography is uncertain. Hence, the
rationale for our randomized trial. Should AI prove as accurate or more ac-
curate in detecting breast cancer, while simultaneously reducing the consid-
erable workload associated with purely human interpretation of screening
mammograms, it would represent a significant advance in improving quality
of care and efficiency of care for women for whom screening mammography is
routinely recommended. (164 words)

Suggested Response

First, this introduction is too wordy and redundant. The last part of the
sentence ("for women for whom screening mammography is routinely
recommended") is unnecessary. After all, the paper is about screening mammography, so ending with "quality of care and efficiency of care" is reasonable.
There are many other targets for trimming you might come up with. More importantly, the general order of sentences doesn't follow the recommendations
in this book. The introduction should start as general as possible and become
more specific, ending with what is to be accomplished to answer the key research question or questions. "Breast cancer is a significant public health
problem" is a good starting point.

I rearranged and trimmed the introduction to come up with the following:

Screening mammography is recommended for detection of breast cancer,
a significant public health problem. Interpreting screening mammograms
is both burdensome and associated with error. Artificial intelligence (AI) is
promising for improving accuracy and efficiency of thoracic, brain, and other
imaging. Its usefulness in screening mammograms is uncertain. Should AI
prove as accurate or more accurate and more efficient than interpretation
by radiologists of mammograms, it would represent a significant advance in
improving quality and efficiency of care. We compared an AI-supported system
to the current practice of double reading by radiologists. (92 words)

The revised introduction includes all the basic elements of the original,
without redundant and unnecessary phrases. There is no need to mention that
a randomized trial was carried out. That will certain become apparent in the
methods section or may have even been included in the title.

Exercise #2

Methenamine hippurate is a urinary antiseptic used to prevent urinary tract infections (UTIs) among women with recurrent infections. It has been compared to the antibiotic nitrofurantoin in a randomized trial. Here is an excerpt from the draft methods section of a paper based on the trial. Your task is to identify what's wrong with the excerpt:

> *Women with recurrent UTIs were randomized in a 1:1 ratio to receive either daily methenamine hippurate (MH) or nitrofurantoin 50 mg daily for a period of 12 months, with the primary outcome being the self-reported incidence of UTI over the 12-month period. Ours was an open-label trial. Recurrent UTI was defined as having three or more UTIs diagnosed in a clinical setting in the preceding 12-month period. Eligible participants were also at least 18 years of age, were not taking antibiotics at the start of their participation, and did not have known immunodeficiency or structural abnormalities or other conditions that increased the risk of UTI. Use of formaldehyde-containing preparations was also an exclusion criterion.*

Suggested Response

The paragraph above is problematic in many ways, but the overarching problem is that it ignores one of the 5Cs—consistency. The methods section should be organized systematically. I based the excerpt on an actual study that appeared in 2022 in the *British Medical Journal*[1] (https://www.bmj.com/content/376/bmj-2021-0068229.long). You can see that the methods section for this article is organized into study design, participants, randomization and masking, procedures, outcomes, statistical analysis, and patient and public involvement. Always follow a suitable design when writing your methods section. While the excerpt doesn't include all methods, descriptions of the participants are scattered among other information. Instead, the women's age, past history of UTI, and exclusions should all be described in one category together.

To many readers, the mention of formaldehyde might be perplexing. Methenamine hippurate is converted to formaldehyde in the urine and has

---

[1] Harding C, Mossop H, Homer T, et al. Alternative to prophylactic antibiotics for the treatment of recurrent urinary tract infections in women: Multicentre, open label, randomised, non-inferiority trial. BMJ 2022;376:e068229. doi:10.1136/bmj-2021-0068229

an antiseptic effect. This may have been mentioned in the introduction of the paper, but if not, an explanation should be included in the methods section, such as:

MH is converted to formaldehyde in the urine, which has antiseptic properties. Use of formaldehyde-containing medications was therefore also an exclusion criterion.

Starting with a standard framework such as the one that appears in the actual BMJ article will help you organize your methods so that they are clear and complete.

Exercise #3

A researcher has recently completed a survey of parents about their thoughts about their children receiving prescription opioid medications for orthopedic surgery. The ClinicalTrials.gov record number is NCT05344118.[2] Your task is to find the results of the study and summarize the most important of them.

Suggested Response

The results are easily found by clicking on the "Results Posted" tab for the study record in ClinicalTrials.gov.

This is a cross-sectional survey study, so there isn't a need for a flow diagram. Parents of children undergoing orthopedic surgery were simply surveyed. It's helpful to provide an overview of the characteristics of the parents surveyed, all of which you can find by scrolling to the bottom of the results page including the outcomes tables. This simple paragraph is enough:

125 parents/guardians completed the survey (88 mothers, 26 fathers, 5 grandparents, 4 legal guardians, and 2 who did not specify their relationship to the child). 103 (82.4%) of the respondents were white, 13 (10.4%) were African American, and the remainder belonged to other racial or ethnic groups or more than one group, or did not specify their race or ethnicity. 81 (64.8%)

---

[2] "Parental perceptions on prescription opioid use for pain control in children undergoing orthopedic surgery," principal investigator Joseph D. Tobias, MD.

were married. 85 (69.7%) were employed, and 39 (32.2%) had a college degree or higher level of education.

You can use your discretion about whether to include the high proportion who spoke English at home. The survey was administered in English and non-English-speaking parents were excluded (which is specified under the "Study Details" tab), so I don't think the very high proportion of those who spoke English at home is worth including as a result. Whether and how the gender of the child of the responding parent is relevant isn't clear, and I wouldn't bother describing this among baseline characteristics of respondents, nor would I describe the mean age of the child of respondents.

Turning next to the outcomes, it's difficult to decide what a "primary outcome" would be for a survey study, but the first two results listed appear to be the most important and can be easily summarized with two sentences:

84 (67.2%) of the respondents felt comfortable with their child receiving opioids <u>during</u> surgery; 36 (28.8%) were comfortable but had concerns; and 5 (4%) were not comfortable. 69 (55.2%) of the respondents felt comfortable with their child receiving opioids <u>after</u> surgery; 45 (36%) were comfortable but had concerns; and 11 (8.8%) were not comfortable.

Parents were asked additional questions about the safety of opioids and safe storage, etc., as well as how informed they believed they were. You could include their self-assessed opioid education as a baseline characteristic rather than an outcome. I believe it's better considered to be an outcome of the research since one purpose of the survey might be to identify gaps in knowledge or education. You could summarize additional responses in a short table, preceded by a short sentence such as, "*Additional responses are summarized in Table 1.*" The challenge would be that the response categories vary among the questions (e.g., yes/no, no education/somewhat informed/very informed). It's therefore easier simply to summarize additional key results in a separate paragraph:

Eighty-one (66.4%) of the parents felt opioids were dangerous. Sixty-eight (54.4%) considered themselves to be somewhat informed about opioids and 45 (36.0%) considered themselves to be very informed. When asked about safe storage of opioids, 40 (57.4%) believed a locked place was best; 45 (36.9%) responded that they should be stored out of reach of children. [This result is a bit perplexing, since I believe "out of reach of children" and in "a locked place" are not mutually exclusive. Nevertheless, the task is to summarize rather than scrutinize the results.] *Forty-five (36.6%) believed it was best to dispose of opioids by taking them to a medical facility, 55 (44.7%) believed it was best to take them to a disposal box or collection event, and 16 (13.0%) felt it was best to flush them down a drain/toilet.*

Exercise #4

Each of the following statements appears in the discussion section of a paper describing the results of a clinical trial comparing a new anticoagulant medication (solitaban) to an older anticoagulant medication (dabigatran) and to aspirin for the prevention of recurrent stroke (i.e., secondary prevention). Which one statement doesn't belong in the discussion? Why?

1. We found solitaban significantly more effective in preventing recurrent stroke over a 48-month period than either dabigatran or aspirin.
2. The incidences of stroke in the dabigatran and aspirin groups were comparable to those reported by Larsen et al.
3. Based on our results, we believe solitaban is also more effective than apixaban for secondary stroke prevention.
4. An important limitation of our work is the relatively young median age (63) of our study population. The relative effectiveness of solitaban in an older population is unknown.

Suggested Response

Statement 1 is a succinct summary of the main finding of the study and belongs in the discussion. Statement 2 compares one of the key results to a prior study and is also appropriate for the discussion. Discussing limitations of the study, as in Statement 4, is also appropriate. Statement 3 is problematic because the research team did not study solitaban versus apixaban. Their belief in solitaban's greater effectiveness is speculative and is not based on their results. The claim might have been included because the benefit of solitaban in the study was greater than the benefit of apixaban in other studies. However, since a direct comparison wasn't made, the statement is not appropriate. A more appropriate statement might be a call for a future study comparing solitaban to apixaban.

Exercise #5

Peripheral arterial disease is a painful and disabling condition that limits walking. Here is a news story entitled "Over-the-Counter Supplement Improves Walking for Peripheral Artery Disease Patient.[3]" Your task is to construct a 100-word structured abstract based on the story. Clearly, much information about the study is missing, but don't worry about finding additional detail from other sources.

The over-the-counter supplement nicotinamide riboside, a form of vitamin B3, increased the walking endurance of patients with peripheral artery disease, a chronic leg condition for which there are few effective treatments.

In a preliminary, randomized, double-blind clinical trial led by Northwestern University and University of Florida scientists, patients who took nicotinamide riboside daily for six months increased their timed walking distance by more than 57 feet, compared to participants who took a placebo. As expected, walking speed declined in those who took a placebo, because peripheral artery disease causes progressive declines in walking performance.

"This is a signal that nicotinamide riboside could help these patients," said Christiaan Leeuwenburgh, Ph.D., a UF professor of physiology and aging and senior author of the clinical trial report. "We are hoping to conduct a larger follow-up trial to verify our findings."

The scientists recruited 90 people with an average age of 71 who had peripheral artery disease, or PAD, to test the effects of nicotinamide riboside. The supplement is increasingly popular as an anti-aging treatment—sales exceeded $60 million in 2022 in the U.S. alone—but there has been scant evidence of any benefit in healthy people. Nicotinamide riboside is a precursor for the essential compound NAD, which plays roles in the body related to energy generation, improved blood flow, and DNA repair.

Because PAD is associated with problems generating energy within muscle cells, McDermott and Leeuwenburgh thought that nicotinamide riboside, by improving energy generation, could help improve walking in people with the disease.

And, indeed, that's what they found. Participants taking the supplement walked an average of 23 feet more in a six-minute walking test after six months, while those taking a placebo walked 34 feet less. Those who took

---

[3] https://news.ufl.edu/2024/06/peripheral-artery-disease-supplement/. Accessed 29 April 2025.

*at least 75% of the pills they were supposed to take performed even better,
adding more than 100 feet to their walking distance, compared to people who
took a placebo.*

*(The researchers also tested if resveratrol, a compound best known for being
in red wine, could boost the effects of nicotinamide riboside; they found no additional benefits.)*

*PAD affects more than 8.5 million Americans over the age of 40. Caused by the
buildup of fatty deposits in arteries, and associated with diabetes and smoking,
the disease reduces blood flow to the limbs, especially the legs. Walking often
becomes painful, and the disease typically causes declines in walking ability
over time. Supervised walking exercise is first-line therapy for PAD, but most
people with the condition do not have access to supervised exercise.*

*In addition to a larger trial focused on patients suffering from PAD,
Leeuwenburgh hopes to test the effects of nicotinamide riboside on walking
performance in healthy older adults.*

*"We need to test it on a healthy older population before we recommend
healthy people take it," he said.*

Suggested Response

This isn't an easy exercise, partly due to the 100-word limit. Also, not only are
some important details about the study missing, but relevant information is
sprinkled throughout the news story. Start by using the headings background
or aim, methods, results, and conclusions/implications, and insert what information is available. Here's what I came up with:

Background: *PAD causes pain during walking. Supervised exercise helps but is
inaccessible to many. Nicotinamide riboside (NR) is a precursor to a compound
that boosts energy, blood flow, and DNA repair.*

Methods: *90 patients with PAD were randomized to NR or placebo.*

Results: *After 6 months, NR patients walked 23 feet more than baseline in a 6-
minute test; placebo subjects walked 34 feet less. NR patients who took at least
75% of pills walked 100 feet more than baseline.*

Conclusion: *NR is promising in improving walking in PAD. Future studies could
include a larger sample or patients without PAD.* (99 words)

Exercise #6

Review this abstract from the 2010 study about exercise as an adjunctive treatment for insomnia among older adults.[4] Your task is to construct an abbreviated specific aims page of roughly 200 words that could have been used to seek funding for the study. Don't worry about adding citations. Include only one specific aim.

> <u>Objective</u>: *To assess the efficacy of moderate aerobic physical activity with sleep hygiene education to improve sleep, mood and quality of life in older adults with chronic insomnia.*

> <u>Methods</u>: *Seventeen sedentary adults aged > or =55 years with insomnia (mean age 61.6 [SD±4.3] years; 16 female) participated in a randomized controlled trial comparing 16 weeks of aerobic physical activity plus sleep hygiene to non-physical activity plus sleep hygiene. Eligibility included primary insomnia for at least 3 months, habitual sleep duration <6.5h and a Pittsburgh Sleep Quality Index (PSQI) score >5. Outcomes included sleep quality, mood, and quality of life questionnaires (PSQI, Epworth Sleepiness Scale [ESS], Short-form 36 [SF-36], Center for Epidemiological Studies Depression Scale [CES-D]).*

> <u>Results</u>: *The physical activity group improved in sleep quality on the global PSQI (p<.0001), sleep latency (p=.049), sleep duration (p=.04), daytime dysfunction (p=.027), and sleep efficiency (p=.036) PSQI sub-scores compared to the control group. The physical activity group also had reductions in depressive symptoms (p=.044), daytime sleepiness (p=.02) and improvements in vitality (p=.017) compared to baseline scores.*

> <u>Conclusion</u>: *Aerobic physical activity with sleep hygiene education is an effective treatment approach to improve sleep quality, mood and quality of life in older adults with chronic insomnia.*

Suggested Response

Remember that the specific aims page is designed to grab reviewers' attention and to be as impactful as possible. Here's an example of how to start based on what can be inferred from the abstract:

[4] Reid KJ, Baron KG, Lu B, et al. Aerobic exercise improves self-reported sleep and quality of life in older adults with insomnia. Sleep Med 2010 Oct;11(9):934–940. Epub 2010 Sep 1. doi:10.1016/j.sleep.2010.04.014

Insomnia has a significant impact on the mood and overall quality of life of older adults.

Next, we can describe what is known about the problem based on the abstract:

Improving sleep hygiene through education is a useful strategy to alleviate insomnia.

A sentence about what is unknown (the critical gap), and another about the importance of filling it, comes next:

Exercise has many benefits for older adults, but its effectiveness in relieving insomnia as a complement to sleep hygiene education is unknown. As insomnia is a common problem among older adults, assessing the impact of exercise, which has many overall benefits, as an adjunctive therapy is important.

A short solution about the solution to be evaluated comes next:

Our goal was to evaluate the impact of a formal exercise program on insomnia among adults age ≥ 55.

The overarching hypothesis comes next:

We hypothesize that exercise complemented by sleep hygiene education will have more impact than sleep hygiene education alone.

The specific aim for the study is relatively straightforward:

Specific Aim: *To compare the impact upon insomnia of an aerobic exercise program plus sleep hygiene education to sleep hygiene education alone among adults age ≥ 55 years in a randomized trial.*

There is no need to describe study subject eligibility in additional detail, especially given the 200-word limit for the exercise.
A precise hypothesis is needed.

We hypothesize that subjects in the sleep hygiene + exercise group will experience greater improvements in sleep quality, mood, and quality of life than subjects in the sleep hygiene alone group.

Had we more information than what is available in the abstract, we could have included precise numbers about the expected improvements in the Pittsburgh Sleep Quality Index, etc. For the purpose of this short exercise, the hypothesis above is adequate.

Finally, a short sentence on the overall impact of the research is needed:

Should the aerobic exercise program prove effective in enhancing the effect of sleep hygiene education, it will represent a useful tool for addressing insomnia among older adults.

Let's put it all together:

Insomnia has a significant impact on the mood and overall quality of life of older adults. Improving sleep hygiene through education is a useful strategy to alleviate insomnia. Exercise has many benefits for older adults, but its effectiveness in relieving insomnia as a complement to sleep hygiene education is unknown. As insomnia is a common problem among adults, assessing the impact of exercise, which has many overall benefits, as an adjunctive therapy is important. Our goal was to evaluate the impact of a formal exercise program on insomnia among adults age $\geq$ 55. We hypothesize that exercise complemented by sleep hygiene education will have more impact than sleep hygiene education alone.

Specific Aim: *To compare the impact upon insomnia of an aerobic exercise program plus sleep hygiene education to sleep hygiene education alone among adults age $\geq$ 55 years in a randomized trial.*

We hypothesize that subjects in the sleep hygiene + exercise group will experience greater improvements in sleep quality, mood, and quality of life than subjects in the sleep hygiene group.

Should the aerobic exercise program prove effective in enhancing the effect of sleep hygiene education, it will represent a useful tool for addressing insomnia among older adults. (198 words)

Exercise #7

Here is the abstract for a paper that describes a randomized trial of exercise for hip arthritis.[5] Your task is to construct, in no more than 75 words,

[5] Krauß I, Steinhilber B, Haupt G, et al. Exercise therapy in hip osteoarthritis—a randomized controlled trial. Dtsch Arztebl Int 2014 Sep 1;111(35-36):592–9. doi:10.3238/arztebl.2014.0592. PMID: 25249361; PMCID: PMC4174683.

a significance and impact paragraph that could form the foundation for a longer significance and impact statement for a grant application.

Background: *Roughly one in ten persons in the industrialized world suffers from hip osteoarthritis, a disease for which there is no cure. The goal of conservative therapy is to relieve symptoms, preferably with methods that let patients assume responsibility for their own treatment, e.g., physical training.*

Method: *In a randomized controlled trial, we studied the effectiveness of twelve weeks of exercise therapy in patients with hip osteoarthritis (THüKo), compared to no treatment (control group) and placebo ultrasound treatment of the hip (placebo ultrasound group). The primary endpoint was a comparison of the pain scores of the intervention versus control groups on the generic SF-36 health questionnaire. Secondary endpoints included comparisons across all three study groups of scores on the 7 other scales of the SF-36 and on the pain, physical function, and stiffness scales of the osteoarthritis-specific WOMAC Index. The statistical analysis was performed with ANCOVA, with baseline values as a covariate. Between-group effects were subsequently tested pairwise (two-tailed t-tests, alpha = 0.05).*

Results: *As for the primary endpoint, pain reduction was significantly greater in the intervention than in the control group (mean difference 5.7 points, 95% confidence interval [CI] 0.4–11.1 points, p = 0.034). The comparisons across all three study groups (i.e., secondary endpoints, with 71 subjects in the intervention group, 68 in the control group, and 70 in the placebo group) revealed no significant between-group effects with respect to the SF-36. On the WOMAC Index, however, statistically significant differences were found for pain reduction between the intervention and control group (mean difference 7.4 points, 95% CI 3.0–11.8, p = 0.001) and between the intervention and placebo group (mean difference 5.1 points, 95% CI 0.7–9.4, p = 0.024). Comparable mean differences were also found for functional improvement.*

Conclusion: *Twelve weeks of exercise therapy in hip osteoarthritis patients of normal vitality reduced pain and improved physical function. No significant improvement was found in these patients' general health-related quality of life.*

Suggested Response

Let's start with a description of the seriousness of the problem. Fortunately, the first sentence of the abstract provides just such a starting point:

About 10% of people suffer from hip osteoarthritis.

Next, you can discuss what we know about conservative treatment, which is also included in the first paragraph of the abstract:

Conservative treatment is used to relieve symptoms. This includes exercise therapy.

Now that you've covered what is known, it's time to turn to what is unknown:

It is unknown, however, how effective exercise therapy is in relieving pain, physical function, and stiffness.

You can now insert the goal of the research:

Our goal was to compare 12 weeks of exercise therapy to no treatment and placebo ultrasound treatment for hip osteoarthritis.

A short sentence on impact concludes the paragraph:

Should exercise therapy prove effective in reducing pain and quality of life, it can be widely recommended and implemented, providing a useful treatment strategy.

Putting it all together you have:

About 10% of people suffer from hip osteoarthritis. Conservative treatment is used to relieve symptoms. This includes exercise therapy. Our goal was to compare 12 weeks of exercise therapy to no treatment and placebo ultrasound treatment for hip osteoarthritis. Should exercise therapy prove effective in reducing pain and quality of life, it can be widely recommended and implemented, providing a useful treatment strategy. (63 words)

Clearly there is a great deal of detail missing about the type of exercise, etc., but these five sentences can form a framework upon which to add relevant significance and impact details.

Exercise #8

Here is an abstract for a study of shared knowledge among patients with heart failure and caregivers (e.g., spouses, children) and patient self-care behaviors.[6] Your task is to construct a short outline for an approach section that includes brief descriptions about what would fit under specific subheadings.

Background: Patients' knowledge about heart failure (HF) contributes to successful HF self-care, but less is known about shared patient–caregiver knowledge.

Objectives: The purpose of this analysis was to: 1) identify configurations of shared HF knowledge in patient–caregiver dyads; 2) characterize dyads within each configuration by comparing sociodemographic factors, HF characteristics, and psychosocial factors; and 3) quantify the relationship between configurations and patient self-care adherence to managing dietary sodium and HF medications.

Methods: This was a cross-sectional study (N=114 dyads, 53% spousal). Patient and caregiver HF knowledge was measured with the Atlanta Heart Failure Knowledge Test. Patient dietary sodium intake was measured by 3-day food record and 24-hour urine sodium. Medication adherence was measured by Medication Events Monitoring System caps. Patient HF-related quality of life was measured by the Minnesota Heart Failure Questionnaire; caregiver health-related quality of life was measured by the Short Form-12 Physical Component Summary. Patient and caregiver depression were measured with the Beck Depression Inventory-II. Patient and caregiver perceptions of caregiver-provided autonomy support to succeed in heart failure self-care were measured by the Family Care Climate Questionnaire. Multilevel and latent class modeling were used to identify dyadic knowledge configurations. T-tests and chi-square tests were used to characterize differences in sociodemographic, clinical, and psychosocial characteristics by configuration. Logistic/linear regression were used to quantify relationships between configurations and patient dietary sodium and medication adherence.

[6] Bidwell JT, Higgins MK, Reilly CM, et al. Shared heart failure knowledge and self-care outcomes in patient–caregiver dyads. Heart Lung 2018 Jan–Feb;47(1):32–39. doi:10.1016/j.hrtlng.2017.11.001. Epub 2017 Nov 15. PMID: 29153759; PMCID: PMC5722704.

Results: Two dyadic knowledge configurations were identified: "Knowledgeable Together" (higher dyad knowledge, less incongruence; N=85, 75%) and "Knowledge Gap" (lower dyad knowledge, greater incongruence; N= 29, 25%). Dyads were more likely to be in the "Knowledgeable Together" group if they were White and more highly educated, if the patient had a higher ejection fraction, fewer depressive symptoms, and better autonomy support, and if the caregiver had better quality of life. In unadjusted comparisons, patients in the "Knowledge Gap" group were less likely to adhere to HF medication and diet. In adjusted models, significance was retained for dietary sodium only.

Conclusions: Dyads with higher shared HF knowledge are likely more successful with select self-care adherence behaviors.

Suggested Response

You should start with an overview of the research methods, with a numbered heading such as C.1. You can include a sentence such as, "To gain insight into shared HF knowledge, we will administer the Atlanta Heart Failure Knowledge Test to patient–caregiver dyads." The abstract includes a number of variables such as patient and caregiver depression, and patient HF-related quality of life, along with the dependent or outcome variables of management of dietary sodium and HF medications. A short overview paragraph could take this form:

C.1. Overall Strategy: To gain insight into shared HF knowledge, we will administer the Atlanta Heart Failure Knowledge Test to patient–caregiver dyads. We will also collect a number of baseline variables from our study participants, including HF-related quality of life, caregiver health-related quality of life, patient and caregiver depression, and patient and caregiver perceptions of caregiver-provided autonomy support to succeed in HF self-care. We will compare knowledge and self-care behaviors (management of dietary sodium and medications) for the study sample, including differences based on sociodemographic, clinical, and psychosocial variables.

You don't need to list all the data to be collected, nor the specifics of questionnaires, etc. in the overall strategy paragraph. The paragraph is simply designed to give reviewers an overview of what will be accomplished so they have a frame of reference as they read more details in the rest of the approach section.

Next, you can describe the first aim. The first aim can include not only the knowledge test but also collection of the various baseline variables described in the abstract:

C.2. Specific Aim #1: *To identify heart failure (HF) knowledge among patient–caregiver dyads, and to identify differences in knowledge based on demographic, clinical, and psychosocial characteristics of patients and caregivers.*

Notice that the aim is quite descriptive. You can include a hypothesis to accompany the aim or, alternatively, simply state in general terms how the aim will be accomplished. A hypothesis could take this form:

We hypothesize that patient–caregiver dyads with higher levels of HF knowledge will include both patients and caregivers with higher quality of life, lower rates of patient and caregiver depression, and higher patient and caregiver perception of autonomy support for HF self-care.

To describe how the aim will be accomplished, you could state:

We will administer the Atlanta Heart Failure Knowledge Test to patient–caregiver dyads as well as tools to measure patient and caregiver quality of life, patient and caregiver depression, and patient and caregiver perception of caregiver-provided autonomy support for self-care.

Under the aim, you can provide more details about the tools to be administered, recruitment of participants, and who will complete the test and questionnaire and how. You can describe the statistical analyses for comparison of knowledge to other variables here or in a separate statistical analysis section that covers both aims. The more detail you can squeeze in, the better.

For a second aim, consider:

C.3. Specific Aim #2: *To compare HF knowledge to self-care behaviors.*

This aim should be accompanied by a hypothesis, such as:

We hypothesize that greater knowledge is associated with better sodium and medication management, and that self-care is also influenced by sociodemographic, clinical, and psychosocial variables.

The second aim is written to describe not only the relationship between knowledge and self-care but also the influence of the other variables to be collected. Keep in mind that you don't know the results of the study as you write your approach. Thus, you don't know if some of the variables to be collected influence knowledge, which in turn influences self-care, or if they have an independent influence. Take caregiver depression, for example. It may influence knowledge, but two dyads with equally poor knowledge might have poorer self-care behaviors if one of the caregivers is depressed.

Again, lots of detail is needed under C.3., which can be placed under headings such as C.3.1, C.3.2, etc. You need to describe the tools used to measure sodium and medication management, and how the comparison will be made. You can include details about statistical analysis for this comparison here or in a separate section.

A statistical analysis section (including power and sample size) can be put under heading C.4. It could include the specific methods described in the abstract, including multilevel and latent class modeling, regression, etc. Who will complete these procedures, how, and when should be described. A power and sample size calculation is almost always a good idea. In this example, the abstract includes categories or "configurations" for higher and lower knowledge. Estimates for the differences in self-care behaviors based on these two categories could be used to determine how many patients are required for the study.

You can use an additional subheading (C.5) for sections on challenges, limitations, and alternative strategies. These challenges could include encouraging patients and caregivers to complete the various questionnaires (a financial incentive could help), etc. A subheading for a timeline of activities could be included, as well as another for dissemination activities (e.g., conference presentations and manuscripts).

Exercise #9

Here is the first part of an abstract published in the journal *Molecular Aspects of Medicine* about the role of the microbiota in the development and progression of glaucoma.[7] Your task is to convert the passage to a version no more than 100 words long suitable for non-experts with roughly a high school education. Feel free, of course, to search online or elsewhere for definitions of terms with which you might not be familiar.

---

[7] Huang L, Hong Y, Fu X, et al. The role of the microbiota in glaucoma. Mol Aspects Med 2023 Dec;94:101221. doi:10.1016/j.mam.2023.101221. Epub 2023 Oct 21. PMID: 37866106.

Glaucoma is a common irreversible vision loss disorder because of the gradual loss of retinal ganglion cells (RGCs) and the optic nerve axons. Major risk factors include elder age and high intraocular pressure (IOP). However, high IOP is neither necessary nor sufficient to cause glaucoma. Some non-IOP signaling cascades can mediate RGC degeneration. In addition, gender, diet, obesity, depression, or anxiety also contribute to the development of glaucoma. Understanding the mechanism of glaucoma development is crucial for timely diagnosis and establishing new strategies to improve current IOP-reducing therapies. The microbiota exerts a marked influence on the human body during homeostasis and disease. Many glaucoma patients have abnormal compositions of the microbiota (dysbiosis) in multiple locations, including the ocular surface, intraocular cavity, oral cavity, stomach, and gut. Here, we discuss findings in the last ten years or more about the microbiota and metabolite changes in animal models, patients with three risk factors (aging, obesity, and depression), and glaucoma patients.

Suggested Response

Knowing how to start a paragraph for non-experts is the first challenge, given that, unlike in a clinical trial, there isn't a clear "bottom line" result to emphasize first. There are two terms that should probably be defined: glaucoma and microbiota. Two opening sentences could include these definitions:

The microbiota is micro-organisms (bacteria and viruses) that live on or in different body parts such as the mouth, stomach, and intestines and on and inside the eye. Glaucoma is an eye disease in which nerves break down and vision is lost.

Next, you can talk about what else is known based on the abstract excerpt:

Important risks for glaucoma include older age and increased pressure in the eye. Other risks include gender, diet, obesity, depression, and anxiety. We know the microbiota has a big impact on many diseases.

You can next include the purpose of the review paper described in the abstract excerpt:

We review findings over the last 10 years about the microbiota and glaucoma.

I don't think a further description of the studies (e.g., animal studies) is needed for a piece for non-experts.

An impact statement can end the paragraph:

Better understanding of how glaucoma develops will help us develop new treatments.

Putting it all together:

The microbiota is micro-organisms (bacteria and viruses) that live on or in different body parts such as the mouth, stomach, and intestines and on and inside the eye. Glaucoma is an eye disease in which nerves break down and vision is lost. Important risks for glaucoma include older age and increased pressure in the eye. Other risks include gender, diet, obesity, depression, and anxiety. We know the microbiota has a big impact on many diseases. We review findings over the last 10 years about the microbiota and glaucoma. Better understanding of how glaucoma develops will help us develop new treatments. (99 words)

The Flesch–Kincaid grade level (checked in Microsoft Word) is 10.1, which makes the paragraph suitable for the intended audience.

Exercise #10

This final exercise is meant for fun and relates to the Writing for Wellness chapter (Chapter 14). Below is a prompt I created for our Words for Wellness Group:

We got to the "village" quite late, nearly 7 p.m. I looked about but didn't see anything that resembled a real village. There was a rusty tin shack hidden among the slender palms some distance from us. We waited patiently. The elderly man, who had apparently seen us, emerged from the twilight about 20 minutes later and sat down on a tree stump, which looked quite fresh as loggers had been in the area only a few weeks earlier. He had quite a story to tell.

Continue the story by adding 300 words.

Suggested Response

I've introduced this prompt to different groups of writers. The individual responses have been really creative and well written. Some writers have turned the prompt into a story about monsters. Others have described an environmental catastrophe. One writer continued the prompt with the foundation for a children's story. Below is what I came up with:

> *He began speaking without waiting for Lucy, our translator. She had stepped away for a moment. She came back and did her best to translate what she was hearing. His name was Solu and he lived nearby. He and his fellow villagers lived in modest dwellings hidden among the trees. They never cleared any part of the forest to create a village out in the open for fear of what Lucy translated as "enemies," and which we understood to be rival tribes. Solu's discourse was monotonous. He didn't look at anyone directly, not even Lucy.*
>
> *After a few minutes of describing the village, the local food sources, and after asking to inspect my camera, Solu started to talk about what he had seen. It was gray in color, like an elephant according to Solu, though I couldn't imagine where he had ever seen an elephant. It was roughly the size of a water buffalo, an animal Solu was more likely to have encountered. It was nearly silent as it walked through the village. On this point Solu was especially clear—no roaring or grunting that one might associate with such a vicious animal.*
>
> *Lucy pressed him several times to speculate as to what he had seen. Each time he responded that he had no idea. I looked at him intensely as he raised his eyebrows, a gesture meaning that he was mystified. I thought at the very least Solu had some idea what he had seen. He may even have been completely certain. A rogue bull of some sort?*
>
> *Lucy got frustrated. Solu wouldn't stop long enough to let her translate for us, and we therefore missed much of the story. Eventually he led us into a dense part of the wood in which a bamboo shack was well hidden.*

I supplied the prompt to ChatGPT. Here's what it came up with:

> *The old man squinted at us through the fading light. His face was a maze of wrinkles, each line etched with the weight of years, of stories lived and lost. He didn't say anything at first, just pulled out a small pipe from his tattered coat and lit it, the smoke curling lazily in the warm evening air.*

"I see you came looking," he finally said, his voice raspy but steady. His eyes flickered to the tin shack hidden among the palms, then back to us. "This place, it's not what it used to be. Not a real village anymore, not since the fire."

I exchanged a glance with my companion, the curiosity burning in both of us. Fire? We hadn't heard anything about that. The maps showed a small settlement here, one we hoped to visit for supplies before moving on. But this . . . this was something else.

"Used to be full of life, people, families, children playing near the trees," the old man continued, his voice taking on a distant quality. "But the fire came down from the hills. They tried to stop it, but . . . it took everything. Left nothing but the skeletons of homes and the memories of the ones who lived here."

The shack made sense now, a last remnant of what once was. I noticed the charred trunks of trees around us, their bark blackened as if the land itself had tried to forget.

"And you?" I asked, my voice hushed, unsure if I wanted to know the answer. "Why are you still here?"

He chuckled softly, a dry, humorless sound. "Because someone has to remember." He paused, puffing again at his pipe. "Not all ghosts leave."

I'm curious about which response to the prompt you prefer.

Index